THE
NURSE
As an Individual,
Group, or
Community Consultant

THE
NURSE

As an Individual, Group, or Community Consultant

Frances C. Lange, R.N., M.S.N., D.S.N.
Independent Nurse Consultant
Formerly Associate Professor of Nursing
University of Alabama School of Nursing
University of Alabama in Birmingham
Birmingham, Alabama

APPLETON-CENTURY-CROFTS/Norwalk, Connecticut

0-8385-6992-7

Notice: The author(s) and publisher of this volume have taken care that the information and recommendations contained herein are accurate and compatible with the
standards generally accepted at the time of publication.

Copyright © 1987 by Appleton-Century-Crofts
A Publishing Division of Prentice-Hall

87 88 89 90 91 / 10 9 8 7 6 5 4 3 2 1

Prentice-Hall of Australia, Pty. Ltd., Sydney
Prentice-Hall Canada, Inc.
Prentice-Hall Hispanoamericana, S.A., Mexico
Prentice-Hall of India Private Limited, New Delhi
Prentice-Hall International (UK) Limited, London
Prentice-Hall of Japan, Inc., Tokyo
Prentice-Hall of Southeast Asia (Pte.) Ltd., Singapore
Whitehall Books Ltd., Wellington, New Zealand
Editora Prentice-Hall do Brasil Ltda., Rio de Janeiro

Library of Congress Cataloging-in-Publication Data
Lange, Frances C.
    The nurse as an individual, group, or community
consultant.
    Includes index.
    1. Nursing consultants. 2. Medical consultation.
I. Title. [DNLM: 1. Consultants—nurses' instruction.
2. Nurses. WY 90 L274n]
RT86.4.L36 1987   610.73   86-14139
ISBN 0-8385-6992-7

Cover: Cindy Lee Lombardo
Design: M. Chandler Martylewski

PRINTED IN THE UNITED STATES OF AMERICA

This book is dedicated first and foremost to my husband, Frank, for all his love and support, and especially for his help with the word processor. As he frequently said, he may not be the best secretary, but certainly, the price is right. Special recognition goes to my eldest son, Frank III, and to Billie Rozell, my colleague and friend, for their help in editing this book.

Contents

Preface

This book is intended for use as a basic text for preparing nurse consultants. Both undergraduate and graduate students of nursing who wish to prepare for, or to explore, the possibilities of the nurse consultant role will find the book useful for viewing and assessing the multifaceted components of consulting. Practicing nurses, clinical nurse specialists, public health nurses, school nurses, occupational health nurses, and nursing educators will find it equally valuable as a reference and as a useful basis for evaluating possible consulting activities.

The basic consulting concepts in this book are universal—that is, they are operable in all consulting disciplines. It is the purpose of this book to blend consultation theory, structural stages, consultant intervention strategies, and a theoretical framework with a practical view of the consulting process. The author sees consultation as one of the major ways by which the knowledge and expertise of the professional nurse can be utilized in assisting individual, group, or community clients to cope with problems through better decision making. Thus, the nurse, acting as a consultant in a variety of settings, can be a potent force for effecting planned change.

The four parts of this book are written to promote an understandable and sequential progression of consultation as a very viable and meaningful dimension of the nursing role. Part I, "Introduction to the Consulting Process and the Nurse Consultant Role," explores consultation as a process of collaborative problem solving and client decision making. Chapter 1 introduces the nurse to today's trends in the consulting field, defines consultation, and discusses the educational preparation, skills, and personal characteristics that are essential ingredients in being a successful nurse consultant. Chapter 2 is devoted to a more extensive discussion of the dimensions of the nurse consultant role. The roles of both internal and external nurse consultants are examined and are contrasted, and the newer trend of collaborative internal–external consultation is emphasized. Settings for nursing consultation, and the multiple roles that the nurse consultant fulfills, are also explored in this chapter. Chapter 3 provides an historical overview of the consultation field and includes an in-depth description of a variety of consulting theories pertinent to an understanding of consulting practice.

Part II, "The Consultation Process: Structure, Strategies, and Conceptual Framework," describes an integrating framework for consultation that is easily understood, flexible, and workable. Chapter 4 presents a concise overview of the three progressive phases of the consulting relationship—structural stages, intervention strategies, and a conceptual framework for optimal function—that interact to become the dynamic process of consultation. Chapters 5 through 7 include a breakdown and an in-depth discussion of each phase.

The first phase (Chap. 5) concentrates on the structural step-by-step progression of operational stages that all consulting relations must go through. Knowing how to successfully complete the business of each stage is the primary focus of this chapter.

The special consultant skills that are needed to support the client's goal achievements are the focus of the second phase (Chap. 6). These skills are the intervention strategies that the nurse consultant utilizes so as to facilitate collaboration and a mutually satisfying working relationship between consultant and client.

Effective communication between consultant and client lies in the selection of a framework that delivers a high probability of success. Chapter 7 supplies such a framework for the consultant to use in order to help bridge the gap between theory and practice. Based on a workable approach built from two major, interlocking theories—planned change and decision making—the two models presented in this chapter provide the consultant with the means to communicate meaningfully to the client all important aspects of the consulting process.

Part III, "Nursing Consultation in Action: From Concepts to Reality," illustrates nursing consultation in progress and describes implementations for individual (Chap. 8), group (Chap. 9), and community (Chap. 10) consultation. These chapters are identically structured. Each moves through the stages of the consulting process from entry to termination, with consultant intervention strategies and applications of the theoretical framework supplied throughout. Each chapter is designed to provide the nurse consultant with both a working model and a variety of in-depth examples of individual, group, or community consultations.

Part IV, "Issues in Consultation," focusses on two phenomena that are integral parts of the everyday experiences encountered by the practicing consultant: (1) the ethical issues that pertain to human-relations consulting, and (2) the business issues of marketing, negotiating, and contracting. Chapter 11 is concerned with the ethical and moral responsibilities of the nurse consultant as they affect consulting practice. Issues of conflicting values and ethical decision making (involving such areas as accountability, authority, coercion, confidentiality, fee setting, manipulation, privacy, sexuality, and veracity) are explored in this chapter.

Chapter 12 moves into the area of nurse entrepreneurship and is written primarily for the nurse who will go into consulting as a career; however, it is of equal value to those nurses who "use consultation" as a supplementary activity to their particular nursing roles. The discussions in this chapter on marketing, negotiating, and contracting are designed to bridge the gap between having the desire and expertise needed to be a professional nurse consultant and having the knowledge to get started. This is a "how-to" chapter that will enable the nurse consultant to market skills, negotiate, write contracts, and "get on with" the business of being a successful nurse consultant.

Chapter 13, the final chapter of this book, combines the basic tenets of the consulting process and defines them, using a checklist format. This list of consulting tasks provides a handy reference for the practicing nurse consultant. An additional reference, the Appendix, lists a variety of books that can provide the nurse consultant with additional information on the process of establishing a consulting business.

All queries should be addressed to the author at:

3629 Haven Hill Drive
Birmingham, Alabama 35210

THE
NURSE

As an Individual, Group, or Community Consultant

PART I

Introduction to the Consulting Process and the Nurse Consultant Role

Nursing literature contains very few references to consultation as a nursing role except when viewed as a highly specialized skill. Formal classes in consultation theory are generally taught only to nurses preparing for graduate degrees. Rarely has consultation been viewed as a skill needed by all professional nurses and one that is much more useful than counseling in everyday practice. Consultation, like counseling, is a helping process. While counseling is generally a long-term, intensive, person-oriented bond centered on the exploration of feelings and attitudes, consultation is a task-oriented process based on meeting specified client-identified needs (further clarification and distinctions between counseling and consulting are explored in Chapter 2).

The key word in consulting is collaboration. Collaborating with clients is the most important thing nurses do. In its simplest aspect this involvement means sharing in the solution of an objective problem. Nurses constantly collaborate in the role of nurse consultant with individuals, groups, or larger community organizations to help organize and energize them in their efforts to deal with problems, make decisions, and achieve planned change. Consultation is thus a useful everyday skill for all levels of nursing.

In the past, the consultant has frequently been portrayed as a person who is brought in at the last moment to share the blame for all the mess that has already happened. The consultant has habitually been a management scapegoat or concerned only with organizational functions and staff development. Yet as the roles, responsibilities, and educational status of nurses have grown over the past years, the functional components of the nurse consultant role have also evolved. The practice of consultation in nursing is no longer confined to administrative, educational, and research settings. Today, nurse consultants are utilized in a wide variety of clinical settings, which includes the whole realm of hospital and community organizations as well as all types of local, regional, state, national, and international health-related agencies.

This explosion in consulting activity is stimulating interest among nurses in the identification of what it takes to be a consultant. Certain characteristics do typify the nurse consultant. First, a nurse consultant must have acknowledged expertise in a specific area. Second, the consultant must be able to get things done when not in direct charge of the people concerned. This second characteristic requires knowledge, skill, judgment, and experience in the use of the consulting process. Thus the purpose of Part I is to introduce consultation as a viable role for the professional nurse, and to explore the rationale and requirements for consulting.

CHAPTER 1

Consultation: A Meaningful Skill for the Nurse

Whatever you can, or dream you can, begin it.
Boldness has genius, power and magic in it.

Goethe

In a sense every nurse is a consultant. Some nurses are full-time consultants, many more do consultation part-time or as an extracurricular activity, and all nurses use the consulting process and strategies every day in their nursing activities. Every time a nurse gives advice, information, or assistance based on a choice of alternative actions, the nurse is using consulting techniques. Consultation is more than just an acknowledged expertise in a specialized area. It is a function of the nursing leadership role that encompasses the whole of nursing practice.

Consultants help clients to understand their problems and work with them to make wise decisions. The discharge-planning nurse who offers such post-hospitalization alternatives as nursing home care, ambulatory clinic care, or home health care to a patient or family must also provide them with enough critical information to make a choice. Thus, consultants are catalysts. From the position of acknowledged expertise in a pertinent field of knowledge, the consultant works to acelerate or even create change in situations that might otherwise be overburdened by multiple alternatives, deficient information, or emotional content. Such situations are typically confronted by nursing professionals who are becoming increasingly aware of the value of utilizing the specific skills of the consulting process.

Consultation is rapidly becoming a potent force within the nursing profession and in structured health-related organizations. It is an economical means to increase the technical competence of people in an organization, since consultants typically pass their knowledge on to other people. Thus, from a purely economic standpoint, we are seeing many interesting broad trends in nursing consultation. For example, Kohnke (1978) and Anderson and associates (1985) point out that in the 1970s and 1980s the increased involvement of government agencies in the provision of health services—especially in the areas of quality control, Medicare, Medicaid, rural health, home health care, and the development of ambulatory and community clinics—has greatly increased the demand for professional nursing consultation. Many agencies unable to maintain a technical or clinical specialist on their payroll will call in a nurse consultant for special help or analysis. According to Thorne (1975) and Kirby (1984), the direct hiring of nurse consultants by agencies has recently increased to the point where there are now as many internal consultants employed by health centers, hospitals, health insurance companies, and state or national health agencies as there are independent or self-employed consultants working under contractual agreements.

To be effective as either an internal or external consultant, the nurse must thoroughly understand and apply the various approaches and processes that work in producing planned change. Consultation theory and the strategies of planned change must and can be learned. Expertise comes with continued practice and learning.

DEFINING CONSULTATION

The term "consultation" is used in many different ways. Caplan (1970), Dinha (1980), and Kirby (1984) point out that the term can be applied to almost any professional activity that includes two common elements: (1) solving a designated problem and (2) helping the client improve specific skills or make more effective plans. In addition, consultation has been defined at various times as:

- A two-way interaction—a process of seeking, giving, and receiving help (Lippitt & Lippitt, 1978).
- A process in which the help of the specialist is sought to identify ways to handle work problems involving either the management of clients or the planning and implementation of programs (Caplan, 1970).
- A process involving a set of activities on the part of the consultant that help the client to perceive, understand, and act upon process events that occur in the client's environment (Schein, 1969).
- A process in which a consultant with the requisite knowledge, skills, programs, vision, and methodology helps or influences the client to solve a problem (Egan, 1975).
- A two-way process of seeking, giving, and receiving help (Bell & Nadler, 1985).

The common denominator in the various definitions concerns the fact that consultation is a process of collaborative problem solving and client decision making that can be viewed or structured in a variety of ways. For the purpose of clarity, this book concentrates on a three-way process of interaction that deals with:

1. The developmental sequence of structural stages that take place during the course of consultation.
2. Intervention strategies (planned behavioral actions) used by the consultant.
3. A theoretical framework within which the consultant functions.

Furthermore, the consulting process may be conceived as occurring within a single consulting session or as a series of episodes in an ongoing process. For example, the clinical nurse specialist in cardiac care may conduct a single one-hour consultation session with a staff nurse regarding the care and specialized needs of a surgery patient. In contrast, the educational nurse consultant's task may require repeated visits to a school of nursing as well as multiple consulting sessions with administrative staff, faculty, and nursing students before the school's total curriculum can be fully developed. The primary function of any consultant is to facilitate human potential—that is, to develop the capacity of self-renewal within individuals, groups, or communities seeking help (Lange, 1979). The essential consultant relationship consists of certain key elements as described in a much-quoted, classic article, "Dimensions of the Consultant's Job," written by Ronald Lippitt in 1959:

1. The consultant relationship is a voluntary relationship between
2. a professional helper (consultant) and a help-needing system (client)
3. in which the consultant is attempting to give help to the client in the solving of some current or potential problem
4. and the relationship is perceived as temporary by both parties.
5. Also, the consultant is an "outsider," that is, not a part of any hierarchial power system in which the client is located (p. 5).

With the trend toward internal consultants, Lippitt's fifth element is no longer valid. The internal consultant is now operative as an integral part of the system. Within the organizational setting, the consultant's general concern is to improve the functional capacities of the organization or, more specifically, the supervision, administration, and continuing education level of its staff. Internal consultation emphasizes the leadership role of the consultant, since it provides opportunities to model professional behaviors and to increase the knowledge and skills of the clients.

As a principle, the internal consultant attempts to avoid personal involvement with the client, since this tends to confuse or destroy an effective relationship. Consultation is best used when it guides clients toward productive decision making and provides them with the expertise and collaboration needed to reach their goal. This means that the consultant must function external to the situation while acting within the organization. This concept of internal versus external consultant roles is further explained in Chapter 2.

A collaborative consulting relationship does not imply equal power. In fact, the consultant has no direct power to make changes or implement programs, and any authority to function is given to the consultant by the client for only a temporary period of time. The client is in need of the expertise of the consultant for a specific purpose, but retains the ultimate power of decision making. Thus, power and authority on the part of the consultant are dictated by client needs at any particular point in time. The consultant is employed not to manage but to facilitate. The consultant does not usually receive direct control of a situation but is allowed to participate in and influence that situation.

RATIONALE FOR THE NURSE CONSULTANT ROLE

A more definitive definition of the nurse consultant is spelled out by the Nurse Consultants Association (NCA) in its by-laws as:

> An individual who is a currently licensed registered nurse and uses nursing knowledge and experience to promote optimum health care through media other than direct patient care. This individual may be self employed or work for a health related industry. The work medium may be, but is not limited to education, research, consultation, or product development. The position in which the individual is employed utilizes the knowledge and skill of a professional nurse. (NCA By-Laws, 1984)

The first prerequisite for being a nurse consultant is acknowledged expertise in a specific practice area. Today, more nurses have graduate degrees and specialized areas of practice than at any time in nursing history. The nurse acting as consultant thereby has something to offer in the area of specialized knowledge and expertise.

There is a growing need for nurse consultants based on increased technology, increased longevity of the population, increased specialization among health professionals, and the diversification of health-care settings. We are in the midst of an economic realignment of health services to trim operating costs and promote efficiency. It makes economic sense to hire nurse consultants, on an as-needed basis, to assist in solving problems specific to nursing rather than to maintain a large staff of experts. Also the continued increase of government reporting regulations, such as the Professional Standards Review Organization (PSRO) and Diagnostic Related Groups (DRGs), demands high expertise from many different health disciplines. Consulting and nursing management firms are growing rapidly, large hospitals and medical centers are establishing their own consulting groups, and individual consulting practices are proliferating.

Nurse consultants are now utilized in every field that involves nursing practice, education, administration, and research. The only limitation in consulting is the nurse's imagination. No matter how obvious the solutions to problems might seem, people can use help in solving them and, moreover, they are willing to pay for that help.

Nursing consultation is very often less than a full-time job. It fits well into the lifestyle of many nurse educators, administrators, and clinical specialists. The majority of nurse consultants today, in fact, maintain other positions in the health field as an economic and professional base from which to provide consulting services. On the negative side of consulting, job security depends on personal initiative, effective marketing, and a high level of technical expertise; this means that it is often difficult to achieve financial security from consulting endeavors alone without having first established a reputation within the nursing field. Still, consulting offers many rewards. It is a constant professional challenge. Each new client brings a new problem and the consultant must search for the solution and guide the collaborative problem-solving process to the point of client decision making and action. Consulting brings with it a sense of independence and self-satisfaction unknown to many other roles within the health-care service field.

CHARACTERISTICS OF A CONSULTANT

The successful consultant must possess a degree of mental agility, be highly analytical, and be able to evaluate situations quickly. At the same time, consultation demands excellent communication and social skills. For example, the consultant must be self-confident, sensitive, and receptive, and be able to analyze people without appearing to do so. This requires good listening skills. A consultant must be able to teach without being condescending. Dealing with individual clients as well as administrators, middle management, and staff all in a single setting can be difficult. It demands a forceful yet nonvolatile disposition and a nonjudgmental attitude as mandatory personal characteristics.

Personal and professional skills must be delicately balanced for successful consulting. Expertise as a technical specialist alone will not do it. The consultant must convey an image of integrity and concern, and the social projection of that image is every bit as important as technical skill. Social gatherings appear to be a part of almost every consulting relationship, especially in group situations. Formal dinners, coffee breaks, and informal "buzz" sessions all serve the purpose of clarifying the entire range of involvement of people and purposes concerned in the endeavor.

Not all consulting is exciting and active. Much time is spent in solitude analyzing the relationships, setting priorities, and detailing the next steps to be taken. The consultant must keep careful notes on all aspects of the interaction. Often schedules and budgets must be developed, contracts negotiated, and reports or summarizations filed. There are many technical and business problems to be managed. Good writing skills and the ability to structure and organize work efficiently are the essential tools of an effective consultant.

EDUCATION FOR CONSULTING PRACTICE

The task of the consultant is to assist clients (individuals, groups, or community systems) to better cope with or solve problems within their perceived environment. If this sounds like the usual statement of purpose for nurses, counselors, and teachers, we should not be surprised. The commonalities of service roles are obvious, and the behavior models of each role are frequently intertwined. Although the nurse or teacher may focus on the passing of information, and the counselor on facilitating accurate expressions of thought, values, and feelings, they frequently also take on a consulting role. The consultant combines a wide range of experience and expertise in a specialized field with a full awareness of interpersonal and organizational dynamics so as to make information available in a manner that enhances the problem identification, problem-solving, and resolution skills of the client.

At the present time, the majority of practicing nurse consultants have simply picked up their skills in the course of performing the multiple and related tasks of professional nursing. It is generally assumed that, with experience, the professional nurse prepared as a clinical, educational, or administrative specialist has accrued sufficient knowledge to function as a consultant. However, as already pointed out, the recent demand for nurse consultant services in areas such as program assessment, program development, and program evaluation along with the rapid growth of specialization in nursing care has fostered our recognition of the consultant role as a special field requiring a unique focus and competency for realization. Now, nursing education must work toward developing new programs that can provide a learning base for this new breed of nurse consultant. Courses integrating both the theoretic and leadership approaches, along with courses in small business management and entrepreneurship, need to be specifically designed to indoctrinate the nurse into the consultant role (Anderson et al., 1985). These courses can be part of a master's or doctoral degree program in nursing, or they may be given as a part of a continuing education or staff development program.

Decisions about course content, role behaviors, and proficiency levels needed to be an effective consultant are difficult to make since, according to Froehle (1978) and Naismith (1978), so little empirical data are available regarding the relationship between consultant skill and the desired outcome for the client. It is obvious, however, that to do a good job the nurse consultant needs three kinds of skills, as identified by Dinha (1980), Froehle (1978), and Kirby (1984), among others. These requisite skills are technical, interpersonal, and consulting skills.

Technical Skills

The foundation for consulting skills is specialization and expertise in one or more areas of nursing. If the nurse consultant did not have some expertise the client would not ask for his or her advice. It is only after acquiring some technical expertise that the nurse starts consulting.

Matching consultant expertise with client needs is, at times, a complicated undertaking. Many client–consultant relationships have simply not worked out because of the failure of both consultant and client to make sure that each have the technical competencies needed to function collaboratively. For example, a hospital (client) with a problem involving specific utilization patterns of nurses needs the services of a nurse consultant with a strong background in management and administrative expertise rather than a clinical specialist. On the other hand, the same hospital faced with the problem of updating staff proficiency in direct patient-care situations would need the specific expertise of a clinical specialist–consultant. Dealing with problem areas wherein the consultant fails to identify the real problem or promises to deliver expertise outside of his or her capabilities almost guarantees failure.

Interpersonal Skills

The consultant must have the ability to foster and maintain a helping relationship that facilitates client growth. Included under the generic term of "helping" are all serious informal and formal transactions such as supporting, interviewing, appraising, and counseling.

In a consulting relationship, every interpersonal reaction is a series of learned initiating and responding behaviors—primarily focused on appropriate communication behavior and the effective use of intervention strategies, as discussed in Chapter 6.

The successful consulting relationship according to Kinlaw (1981) is largely a matter of consultants becoming knowledgeable and systematic in their understanding of the helping process and disciplined in the way they conduct themselves.

Additionally, the area of interpersonal relations focuses on and includes such consultant characteristics as trust, openness, flexibility, adaptability, desire to help, honesty with self, and honesty with others.

Consulting Skills

There is a third set of skills that is an essential part of consulting over and above technical expertise and interpersonal skills—these are consulting skills.

Consulting skills are intricately interwoven with the entirety of the consulting process. They involve knowledge of the major consulting theories—planned change and decision making—as well as consultant compentency in the execution of each of the structured, sequential steps or stages involved in any effective consulting endeavor. Successfully completing the business of each stage of the consulting process is the primary focus of this book (the consulting process and related skills are covered in Chapters 4 through 7).

Education for the consultant should thus involve a combination of conceptual and experimental methods. Practical experience and knowledge of the consulting process is supplemented and enhanced by further studies in such academic fields as traditional psychology, behavioral psychology, cultural anthropology, interpersonal and intergroup dynamics, and more particularly, the dynamics affecting personal and social change. Such an educational foundation coupled with an application knowledge of business management skills sets the stage for successful consulting.

The foundations of nursing consultation are broadly based, to say the least. The theoretical course offerings that will benefit a nurse consultant are as diversified as the people and circumstances of the profession. Although consultation, as a client approach, is a valuable adjunct to any nursing activity, nurses planning to do internal or external consulting should prepare themselves in an educationally planned, broad-based program in consultation. Any educational program for the consultant (workshop or formal courses) should include segments of simulated or supervised direct practice as well as study in as many related theoretical fields as is practical or desirable.

All consultant education should include the opportunity for supervised practice. Direct practice consultation should begin with low-demand and low-intensity situations—that is, with consulting techniques applied to dysfunctional aspects that are within the realm of the consultant's knowledge and expertise. Supervision, team practice, and detailed analysis of initial experiences are necessary to enhance learning and to allow the consultant and others to evaluate both personal and professional expertise. The consultant may then move increasingly and confidently to more involved consulting relationships.

THE CLIENT

The word "client" is used throughout this book and denotes the recipient of the consultant's services. The term "consultee" is used only in reference to consulting situations in which the consultant is collaborating with other professionals who are, in turn working with the client. In nursing consultation, we have three types of clients:

- *The individual client* is a one-to-one situation. The individual client can be a patient, family member, nurse, administrator, faculty member, organizational representative, or other professional.

- *The group client* is usually less than ten people in a small, cohesive unit (referred to in this text as a primary group). Examples of group clients include families, unit staff nurses, head nurse groups, and nursing faculties.
- *A community group* is a larger, more diverse, and more complex social system (referred to in this text as a secondary group). The community group is less personal in nature and can include schools, churches, medical centers or large hospitals, community organizations, governmental health agencies, and private foundations.

The Changing Client

In the past, the major employer of nurse consultants has been other nursing organizations or those organizations that employ many nursing personnel, such as hospitals, nursing homes, nursing schools, and agencies involved in direct patient-care situations. Today, the pendulum is swinging toward the utilization of nurse consultants in a much broader range and diversity of human service organizations. Numbered among this group are private and public schools, churches, governmental agencies at all levels, social service agencies, public safety organizations, and even private industries interested in promoting the health interests of their employees.

Generally, two kinds of consultant help are required by human service organizations. The first is assistance in developing or evaluating the provision of health services. Some organizations look only for packaged programs such as health appraisals or health education in specific content areas. The organization usually has a commercial purpose in mind and a singular need for nursing consultation. There is nothing wrong with this type of consultation, but it is usually not very challenging to the consultant.

In the second type, process consultation, the consultant collaborates with the client to jointly review an area of concern, consider the possible causes for the concern, develop a series of potential strategies for intervention, and consider the potential cost–benefit consequences of these strategies; the client then implements the mutually conceived course of action. This approach of process consultation obviously represents the complete professional consulting model, and is explored in greater depth in Chapters 4 through 7.

Choosing a Consultant

When hiring a consultant, the client expects that the consultant will provide the objective, professional advice and guidance required to improve the client's problem situation. Thus, arriving at the decision of when to engage a consultant and choosing who that consultant should be are the client's most important considerations. The timing is generally a function of crisis for the client. The client perceives a problem, present or future, and seeks professional assistance. The client chooses a consultant not only on the basis of the nature of the problem faced but also on the professional qualifications, prior experience, reputation, and recommendations or referrals associated with the consultant.

In choosing a consultant, the client may refer to consultant listings in professional journals. For example, the *Journal of Nursing Administration,* among others, annually publishes a listing of available nurse consultants and details their areas of expertise. Although professional journals do not endorse particular consultants or consultant firms, or even guarantee their effectiveness, they do attempt to provide effective guidelines. However, professional membership does not automatically signify a level of professional achievement.

Consultants are more often hired on the basis of recommendations. Just as the consultant uses his or her personal and professional network to find clients, the client uses a network of business aquaintances to locate a suitable consultant. The client will not hesitate to call the consultant or previous clients for references. All consultants should develop and maintain reference files. "Whenever a client's name is given for reference, alert the client so they can expect the call. As a usual rule, do not ask for written references, but save any letters praising your work. Most people are more willing to spend time on the phone than to write a letter" (Lant, 1985).

The client's final steps in choosing a consultant involve personal contact with the consultant to clarify all objectives and arrangements. This includes the process of negotiating and the signing of a formal contract (see Chapter 12 for a discussion of contracting and for illustrations of sample contracts). Contracting safeguards both the client and the consultant and should always be developed in as much detail as possible.

Consultation is a collaborative relationship and must be approached evenly by both client and consultant. Without exception, the consultant comes on board expecting to do the job in a professional manner. Usually the consultant is confident that his or her skills and experience are sufficient for the task involved; but the consultant cannot be effective without the commitment and cooperation of the client. In the final analysis, the consultant must gain the confidence of the client through demonstrated competence and technical knowledge, and the client gives the consultant the freedom, trust and support as needed to do the job.

SUMMARY

The type of professional identity associated with a consultant has no set structure. It is sometimes difficult for nurses to fit into the consultant role because it is not "doing for others" (the traditional nursing role) but rather helping others "do for themselves." Consulting is never "direct" control. A manager or nursing supervisor is someone who has direct control over the action. A consultant must be willing to stand by with no direct control over anything. The consultant wants only to influence the client and frequently steps out of the picture before successful conclusion of the problem. The key to understanding the nurse consultant role is to understand and be willing to accept the differences between a consultant role and the roles of a super-visor–manager, teacher, or nurse practitioner. There is no power in consulta-tion to enforce behavioral change in others. The optimal relationship between consultant and client is one in which the consultant is perceived to have expertise in both technical and human behavioral areas. Further, this exper-tise must be balanced with a truly collaborative relationship. Within this relationship, the client allows the consultant to provide the leadership neces-sary to explore a given problem situation, and the consultant respects the client's right to make the final decisions.

The education of a nurse consultant is a "mixed bag" of professional expertise, interdisciplinary education, and personal experience. Besides ex-pertise in the nursing discipline, the nurse consultant must have a working knowledge of general psychology, social psychology, communication theory and interpersonal relationships, research, and business administration and finance, to name but a few of the disciplines that relate to the consultant's work. The nurse consultant must rely on a broad educational background, with as much mix as possible, and balance it against enough in-depth train-ing in consulting methodology to achieve a solid academic foundation.

Overall education for the nurse consultant should follow this trend and foster the development of consultant competencies that result in:

1. Increased confidence in consulting ability as a result of practical experiences.
2. Better theoretical framework for consultation.
3. Exploration of personal values directly and indirectly related to consultation.
4. Better understanding of one's own consulting style.
5. Increased understanding of what to expect during consultation.

This first chapter has been an overview of the consulting process and the role of the nurse consultant. For the nurse interested in consultation, consulting skills are learnable skills. There are many positions and opportu-nities for nurses to work as consultants, both inside and outside of health-related organizations. Often what the nurse consultant needs is simply a structure or guideline to follow that will fill in the missing pieces of needed information. This book will help complete the picture of the nurse consul-tant. The concepts and examples presented in this book are applicable to all forms of individual, group, or community consultations. The central premise is to provide a flexible structure of resource material and ideas for the design of consulting activities.

SELECTED REFERENCES

Anderson, R., Fitzpatric, J., & Thurkettle, M. The new breed. *Nursing Success Today,* 1985, *2*(3), 5–8.

Bell, C., & Nadler, L. *Clients and consultants.* Houston: Gulf Publishing Company, 1985.

Caplan, G. *The theory and practice of mental health consultation.* New York: Basic Books, 1970.

Dinha, D. *Consultants and consulting styles.* Vienna, Va.: MCP Publishing Company, 1980.

Egan, G. *The skilled helper.* Monterey, Calif.: Brooks/Cole Publishing Company, 1975.

Froehle, T. Systematic training for consultants through competency-based education. *Personnel and Guidance Journal,* March 1978, 437–441.

Kinlaw, D. *Helping skills.* San Diego: University Associates, 1981.

Kirby, J. *Consultation: The practice for the practitioner.* San Diego: University Associates, 1984.

Kohnke, M. *The case for consultation in nursing.* New York: Wiley, 1978.

Lange, F. The multifaceted role of the nurse consultant. *Journal of Nursing Education,* 1979, *18*(9), 30–34.

Lant, J. *The consultant's kit: Establishing and operating your successful consulting business* (2nd ed.). Cambridge, Mass.: JLA Publications, 1985.

Lippitt, R. Dimensions of the consultant's job. *Journal of Social Issues,* 1959, *15*(2), 5–12.

Lippitt, R., & Lippitt, G. *The consulting process in action.* La Jolla, Calif.: University Press, 1978.

Naismith, D. Educational opportunities and consulting skills. In G. Lippitt & R. Lippitt (Eds.), *The consulting process in action.* La Jolla, Calif.: University Associates, 1978.

Nurse Consultants Association. By-laws, approved March 3, 1984, Colorado Springs, Colo.

Schein, E. *Process consultation: Its role in organizational development.* Reading, Mass.: Addison-Wesley, 1969.

Thorne, M. (Ed.). Introduction. *Health Education Monographs,* winter 1975, *3*(4), 359–361.

CHAPTER 2

Dimensions of the Nurse Consultant Role

Those who think must govern those who toil.
Oliver Goldsmith

Basic dynamics in a consulting situation vary, as do the types of health agencies requiring help and the types of nurse consultants available to provide help. Fundamentally, as mentioned in Chapter 1, there are two major divisions or categorizations of consultants—internal and external. Other terms used for the two categories are generalists and specialists (Lippitt & Lippitt, 1978; Merry & Allerhand, 1977; Stanhope & Lancaster, 1984) and affiliated and independent (Fay, 1985). The internal consultant is the person existing within the organization who is given the responsibility to plan and implement constructive change as an identifiable formal or informal function. Conversely, the external consultant is brought into a situation from outside the organizational setting—that is, as a "hired expert." As a personal part of the organization, the internal consultant has unique potential and a unique set of problems. On the other hand, the external consultant is "wanted," even when imposed on a subsystem client by the organizational leadership, and thus usually enjoys optimal attention and cooperation from the client. The following is a more extensive discussion of the characteristics of internal and external consulting roles.

THE INTERNAL CONSULTANT

In recent years it has been demonstrated by such authors as Bell and Nadler (1985), Kohnke (1978), and Stanhope and Lancaster (1984) that a consultant can be effectively used within the internal organization to deal with such areas as the facilitation of management, staff, and patient problem solving; to administer, design, and conduct training and educational programs; or to fulfill dual roles, such as clinical specialist–consultant. Employing a full-time nurse consultant can be a time-saver for the health agency, since an internal consultant does not require the orientation and briefings that an external consultant must receive prior to any constructive activity. The internal consultant also has the advantage of having a view of the total program and is in a position to recommend and effect changes on many levels.

Since internal consultation is a fairly recent role for the nurse, a major disadvantage is that the role, function, and activities are frequently misunderstood by the employer and other employees and, in some cases, by the consultants themselves. It is vitally important that the ground rules concerning the consultant's role be identified, preferably in writing; that the nurse functioning as an internal consultant be clearly labeled as such; and that the position not require the nurse to function in the dual roles of supervisor and consultant. The role of nurse supervisor should never be conceived as a consultant role, since the term denotes line responsibility and implies a formal power and authority over others that negates the basic collaborative structure vital to all consulting relationships. However, there are instances in which an organization is not large enough to support a full-time internal consultant and the dual role becomes a necessary condition to employment. In such situations, the roles of in-service educator–consultant or clinical specialist–consultant are the most frequent and effective dual role designations, since neither role involves any direct power or authority over other employees. If any lack of understanding of the position and functions of the consultant exists, the full potential of the nurse consultant will not be acknowledged and, as a result, the consultant's effectiveness will not be fully realized. Without a specifically defined job description as well as administrative and staff support, the consultant risks having the consulting process interrupted, delayed, and even destroyed.

The internal consultant typically does not have as much freedom as his or her external counterpart. Like any employee, the consultant has additional responsibilities to the employer. Time and activities must be accounted for; problems that arise must be solved even though the consultant would rather not be involved with the problem; and the internal consultant often suffers from the lack of total objectivity and openness within the consulting setting. Table 1 more clearly identifies the advantages and disadvantages of the role of the internal consultant.

THE EXTERNAL CONSULTANT

The external consultant is a self-employed agent with all the freedom and problems that this entails. External consultants usually operate outside an

TABLE 1. THE ADVANTAGES AND DISADVANTAGES OF THE INTERNAL CONSULTANT ROLE

Advantages	Disadvantages
1. Is more readily available to the client system	1. Is part of the client system and therefore may be part of the problem
2. Salaried position, generally less costly to the client system and pay is not ordinarily tied to results	2. Often able to get by with only "adequate" performance
3. Many benefits, such as health insurance and travel costs, are covered by the employer. No overhead	3. Job is limited. Usually operates at a lower influence level than the external consultant. Help may even be resented by coworkers
4. Knows the language and culture of the client system better	4. May encounter active resistance within the client system because of relationships involving hierarchy, vested interests, and organizational politics
5. Knows the political realities of the client system	5. May be required to assume roles other than those expected of a consultant, such as supervisor or administrative assistant, classroom teacher, troubleshooter, or evaluator. Thus, may suffer lack of objectivity
6. May have a better appreciation of the relative importance of the consultant role in the total plan of the agency	6. Role stress may occur from conflict in defining role expectations and from "role overload." May lack the time to carry out all role obligations

organization's hierarchy. As a result, their influence is indirect and usually only advisory. The external consultant is contracted to complete a specific long-term or short-term task. Payment is strictly negotiable and there are rarely vacations, insurance, social security, or other benefits available.

Certainly, it is not unrealistic for nurses to consider setting up their own private consulting firms. External consulting services usually come under four general headings: health services consulting, educational consulting, administrative consulting, and research consulting. Nursing has a great deal to offer today and consulting is a plausible and desirable occupation for nursing professionals. However, the role of external consultant, like the internal role, has its own advantages and disadvantages that need to be evaluated carefully before entering this type of practice setting. These advantages and disadvantages are summarized in Table 2.

Bell and Nadler (1985) note that internal and external consultants in their ideal form show more similarities than differences; both function as facilitators and resource-persons; both have no direct power or control over implementing the changes needed but instead must depend on others; and both desire to be effective helpers, utilizing the same principles and processes of consultation.

TABLE 2. THE ADVANTAGES AND DISADVANTAGES OF THE EXTERNAL CONSULTANT ROLE

Advantages	Disadvantages
1. Is external to problems within the client system. Has highest impact (influence) on the client system	1. Is an outsider to the client agency. Confusion over authority may present conflict for the consultant and client, especially if the consultant is not clear about his or her role
2. Can negotiate compensation. No limit on earnings or growth potential	2. Pay may be tied to results. Generally viewed as more costly to the client system than internal consultation. Also, the consultant is responsible for all overhead
3. Can choose clients and set own hours as desired (within client limitations)	3. Time given to the client may be limited by a contract that specifies a time factor. There may not be enough time to identify all variables in the situation, and the consultant may meet resistance because the problem remains unidentified
4. Usually is viewed as an expert by those in the client system and is actively sought out	4. Needs more extensive briefing and orientation to the client system
5. Less likely to be caught up in the hierarchy of the system or role confusion. Clients often feel freer to be more open about problems	5. Often does not know all the political realities, language, and other factors of the client system. May not have sufficient time to sort these out

THE NEW TREND: COLLABORATIVE INTERNAL–EXTERNAL CONSULTATION

In large organizations where there are extensive consulting projects to be carried out—such as new program design, staffing patterns and utilization studies, or ongoing program evaluations—there is a trend toward collaborative consultation, or the partnership of internal and external consultants. Here the strengths and weaknesses of each consultant role can be most effectively mobilized and compensated. However, compatibility of the two consultants as individuals is of utmost importance. The best approach is for the internal consultant (rather than the administrator) to take the initiative to locate an external resource-person who possesses the complementary skills needed. According to Margulies (1978) the division of labor for such an inside–outside consultant team is largely self-evident: the outside consultant usually has an easier time requesting and collecting necessary data, while the inside consultant is better able to monitor and follow the collection process. Also, the inside consultant is more effective at marshaling support for feedback sessions, but the outsider is better positioned to make recommendations for innovative risks.

Such teamwork, of course, implies a commitment to cooperation by both consultants, rather than a competitive attitude that frequently arises when a management-hired external consultant is brought into the sphere of influence normally occupied solely by the internal consultant. These types of relationships can be complex, confusing, and competitive, but a working team can handle projects that an individual cannot, and often creates unique and useful combinations of skills.

An internal–external consultant relationship does not always work or guarantee a better final product. For example, a hospital under the direction of a national hospital management organization may have a number of external consultants available as needed or even on a retainer basis. The hospital may suddenly bring in an external consultant without fully informing the internal consultant or without there being sufficient time for communicative interchange between consultants. This situation often results in misunderstanding and resistance, and conditions of high emotional impact can arise. Even the best of internal consultants would be hard put to cooperate fully or deal with their own underlying prejudice. External consultants should be fully aware of any potentially explosive or resistant situation before they enter into it. Careful planning and thorough data-gathering and assessment of any proposed consulting situation is mandatory before contract acceptance.

SETTINGS FOR NURSING CONSULTATION

As noted earlier in this chapter, nurse consultants work with individuals, groups, or communities in four major settings: notably, the management of health services, educational resources, administrative support, and research. No consultant can be a specialist in every field. Therefore, it is important that the nurse enter the field of consultation with a clear idea of the specific services he or she has to offer and of the specific market for those services. Each consultant has different expertise and abilities. The particular area of the consultant's expertise should be analyzed and developed to take advantage of every opportunity for consulting experience. "Research indicates that even the largest consultant firms are emphasizing specialization because it is more marketable and more profitable" (Lant, 1985). This is a major reason for the now popular "team of experts" consulting approach offered by many consulting firms. Expertise is a marketable commodity. Hence, nurses should capitalize on their own unique skills, build and expand these skills, develop a reputation, and improve their marketing techniques (see Chapter 12 for an in-depth discussion of marketing, negotiating, and contracting for consultant services).

Health Services Consulting
The use of consultants for management consultation is an effective way for health-care organizations to handle problems such as improvement of effi-

ciency and effectiveness of patient care, expansion, reorganization, and implementation of evaluation techniques for quality assurance programs.

The consultant role in a health service setting is essentially an elaboration of the skills and expertise appropriate to nursing—that is, advising and collaborating with those who have some influence on, and participation in, the delivery of health-care services. In the broadest sense, this is "expert" consulting because the unique skills and expertise of the consultant are called upon to prescribe for specific problems in specific situations. Such consulting usually assumes that the solution of a problem is due to the client's lack of necessary expertise to solve the problem; and that, with the consultant's help, the client will be able to develop the skills necessary to solve the problem now and in the future.

As previously noted, clinical nurse specialists frequently find themselves in an "expert" consultant role. A few examples of health services consultation by the clinical nurse specialist will help illustrate this condition (drawn from the works of Anders, 1978, and Kohnke, 1978, but not directly quoted).

A staff nurse who encounters a patient with a radical mastectomy and who is unfamiliar or uncomfortable with the postoperative body-image changes produced by such a procedure might request a consultation from an Oncology Clinical Nurse Specialist to determine what techniques and behaviors are needed to deal with the self-image distortions of the patient.

In a cardiac nursing care unit the quality of care given to patients is determined to be below acceptable standards. The Cardiac Nurse Clinical Specialist is the logical consultant to aid the nursing staff in resolving this problem. As an "expert" consultant, the specialist intervenes, choosing from a number of consultant intervention techniques the approach that is best suited to the specific problem.

In another situation, the expert consultant (internal or external) may be used to help staff members more clearly assess and identify problems in a particular nursing unit, even though the staff members are well equipped to handle the daily unit functions. It is common that consistent exposure to a problem area decreases problem identification as well as problem solving, with the end-point being that staff members are "unable to see the forest for the trees." For example, a particular hospital unit may approach the consultant with a request to examine some recent problems that have arisen with an interdisciplinary team approach to patient care that has suddenly "fallen apart" after a successful initial period of implementation. An analysis by the consultant demonstrates that the interdisciplinary team members have been doing their jobs very conscientiously but, in reality, have each been doing their "own thing," with no real communication going on between team members. Time and effort were often duplicated and many patients had three or four history and physical assessment forms on their charts, each done by a separate team member. Under the guidance of the consultant the group readily identifies the problem area as ineffective communication, and sets goals and establishes methods to solve the problem. In this situation, the consultant's expertise is in the area of process consultation—that is, the ability to lead the group through the process stages of problem identification, analysis, the formulation of solutions (decision making), implementation, and evaluation of the solution implemented.

Health services consultants are also in demand by many volunteer community agencies such as the American Lung Association, American Cancer Society, American Red Cross, American Heart Association, and the Visiting Nurse Association. These organizations regularly hire internal and external consultants to collaborate on a multitude of service-oriented projects.

Federal, regional, state, and local governmental agencies such as the Maternal and Child Health Division, Mental Health Associations, and federally funded rural health-care centers employ nurse health service consultants to design, develop, implement, and evaluate specialized services as well as to help staff members become more effective health-care providers.

Educational Consulting

Educational consultation may be utilized for consumer education in a community setting, for staff in-service education in a health agency, and for more formalized levels of educational settings such as public schools or schools of nursing.

The extensive work involved with the accreditation of nursing programs by the National League for Nursing (NLN) and other national, state, regional, and local accrediting bodies has been a major incentive for the use of external educational consultants. The NLN and the regional boards for accreditation of higher education hire nurse consultants to serve on their review boards. Beyond that, nurse consultants are often hired by schools themselves, to assist administration, faculty, staff, and students in preparing for accreditation.

Curriculum planning, design, development, implementation, and evaluation are some of the primary responsibilities of the educational consultant. For example, curriculum development and revision is usually a faculty and administrative group activity, but the nurse consultant provides both with the requisite knowledge to make curriculum decisions and with guidance in the use of that knowledge. Ultimately, the composition of the curriculum is the responsibility of faculty members, but the nurse consultant must provide understanding, explanation, justification, and guidance toward a curriculum compatible with the institutional goals.

Administrative Consulting

Administrative roles in nursing typically require knowledge and abilities not within the scope of the nurse's basic education, and not all nurses currently in administrative positions have this preparation. Even nurse administrators with educational preparation in administrative and managerial skills may encounter organizational problems and issues beyond their capabilities. A nurse consultant with the needed expertise can do much to facilitate the administrator's ability to alleviate the problem. In situations of this kind, the climate is usually very open—that is, the consultant is wanted and the administration is receptive.

However, the consultant may also enter a situation where the climate is not an open one and client hostility may be the early prevailing reaction. This type of consulting taxes the full resources of a consultant. For example, a consultant may be engaged by a hospital administrator who has identified a problem of communication breakdown between the director of nursing and other levels of nursing personnel. The hospital administrator has not been able to intervene in this situation in a positive way, and he or she sees an "out" by hiring a consultant to solve the problem. This is not one of the easier consulting relationships to handle and not all nurse consultants like to work in this type of situation. Here it is difficult to predict success or failure until the consulting relationship is well established. The director of nursing may respond with resistance and anger even though agreeing to be advised. It is easy to see that this particular situation requires a consultant with very special expertise in organizational behavior and human performance. If the consultant cannot feel comfortable in dealing with this type of situation, he or she should not accept the contract, or should withdraw in favor of a consultant who has more expertise in these areas.

Research Consultation

Knowledge of research methodology is essential since the collection and analysis of data is basic to practically all consulting situations (Stevens, 1978). Any consultant involvement in research is most likely to be oriented toward solving practical problems that originate in the actual work environment. It would be an unusual situation for the consultant to be involved in basic (sometimes referred to as "pure") research which is oriented toward describing, explaining, or resolving theoretical problems.

Research activities of the nurse consultant fall generally into two categories. The first involves use of the consultant to direct or actually carry out such activities as needs assessment, community surveys, polling, analysis, and interviews in a variety of settings. As an example, external consultants are often hired to direct community health assessments for urban and rural communities planning primary health-care clinics or specialized health services. In today's market, much of the available federal, state, and private-grant funds are tied to the production of quality research by health agencies. Many agencies, however, do not have the personnel or capacity to formulate and conduct research functions which might qualify for such funds. A nurse consultant with interest and expertise in research matters is often called into educational and service settings to stimulate and help the nursing staff in conducting and interpreting research. Also, with the additional burden of the complicated evaluation mechanisms currently required to report and maintain private or official sources of funding, it is especially difficult for most health services administrators to document the accomplishments of their programs without external consultant help. This inability to document and demonstrate effectiveness and progress caused the demise of many maternal care and primary health care projects that were started in the 1970s and 1980s (Lange, 1983).

The second category of consultant research activities has to do with consultant–client collaboration in the research process itself. Here the research focus is generally on the study of activities that can bring about change in the actual work of social systems. Such activities might include the study of the differences between functional and primary nursing activities with the goal of improving the overall delivery of quality health care.

Additionally, Kohnke (1978) notes that many nurses are interested in participating actively in clinical research but do not have the educational preparation or knowledge to do so. The research consultant is a key person who can assist nurses in the formulation and implementation of pertinent research projects that can stimulate their interest in research and that have the potential, at the same time, to improve their nursing practice.

MULTIPLE ROLES OF THE NURSE CONSULTANT

A major problem facing the nurse consultant today is the multiplicity of roles that he or she is expected to assume. For the nurse, a "position of consultant" is likely to involve not only specific consulting duties but also some functional duties such as leader, expert, coordinator, resource-person, clinical specialist, teacher, or researcher. Such complexity of role, combined with the variety of settings in which the nurse consultant functions, makes it difficult to identify and generalize the roles of a nurse consultant.

It is perhaps easier to view the more obvious roles of the nurse consultant by diagraming them (Fig. 1). In this illustration the nurse consultant is shown as the important component person; the consultant's varied roles provide the skills segment; and his or her effectiveness is depicted as the integration and culmination of the consultant role behavior.

The different roles the nurse consultant may assume call for varying degrees of directive behavior. For example, in some situations the consul-

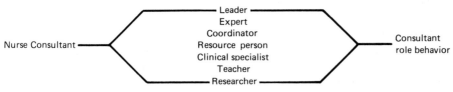

Figure 1. Conceptualizing the roles of the nurse consultant.

tant assumes a leadership posture and initiates activity, while in others the consultant may be a resource-person providing data for the client to use (or refuse) in making decisions. These roles are not mutually exclusive—that is, the nurse consultant may assume any or all of the different roles in a single consulting endeavor.

The majority of the consultant roles have already been mentioned or discussed to some degree and will be further clarified throughout this book. The following section offers a short explanation of each of the roles shown in Figure 1.

Leader

The quality of leadership more than any other single factor determines the success or failure of a consultant. Leadership is an extremely complex interpersonal relationship. As Fiedler and colleagues (1976) point out, "If there is no follower, there is no leader" (p. 2). Members of a group implicitly or explicitly let one person, the leader, make certain decisions and judgments in order to accomplish the group's task.

By virtue of his or her role in assisting and directing others toward goal setting and achievement, the consultant naturally assumes a leadership role. Within the consulting context, leadership is primarily concerned with an informal power that hinges on the interpersonal relationships between consultant and client. As the consulting relationship progresses and the client begins to assume direction, the consultant leadership role undergoes changes. There is no specific "right" style of leadership; what is right is what helps clients achieve their goals. According to Lancaster and Lancaster (1982), a workable concept of leadership takes into account the characteristics and abilities of the leader as well as those of the client, the context or situation in which the leadership takes place, and the quality of the interaction among the participants.

Expert

The expert consultant has unique skills and expertise to deal with a particular problem in a particular situation. Role expertness has as its source the client's belief that the consultant has some information, skill, or ability that can help. Clients normally do not expect the consultant to act directly in their behalf, but they do assume that the consultant possesses answers to the relevant problems or information that will enable clients to come up with their own answers. In any case, clients believe that this information will enable them to reach their goal.

Coordinator

Coordination as defined by Clark and Shea (1979) is synchronization to produce a minimum of conflict and a maximum of collaboration. Coordination can determine the success or failure of a consulting endeavor, since coordination links together the various people and resources, and channels the client activities toward goal achievement. The role of coordinator of change efforts and programs requires the ability to plan, organize, facilitate, energize, manage conflict, and inspire confidence.

Resource Person

A large portion of the consultant's work is connected with knowledge and utilization of resources needed by clients. When working as a resource-person, the consultant usually focuses on three questions: What is needed? Where can it be found? How can it be used?

According to Lippitt and Lippitt (1978), there is a strong tendency on the part of both clients and consultants to do the best they can with what they have at hand, with the result that the information and skills that are needed to do a good job of searching often are lacking or neglected. An even more serious issue exists when a variety of resources are compiled, but without a specific design for utilizing them to arrive at decisions and action plans.

The objective of resource use is to provide relevant information so that the client can make choices from a variety of alternatives. The client has the necessary ability to select and carry out appropriate interventions, but may have insufficient knowledge to recognize what the alternatives are.

Clinical Nurse Specialist

The clinical specialist role of the nurse consultant reflects specialized knowledge, skill, and experience in a particular field. The client hires the consultant to provide a unique service. In the course of providing service to the client, the consultant augments the client's own expertise and potential.

Mary Kohnke (1978), in *The Case for Consultation in Nursing,* stresses the fact that the role of consultant is not new among the functions of the clinical nurse specialist. She further points out the fact that in many clinical nurse specialist situations, the client is frequently another professional nurse (a consultee) seeking consultant help on behalf of a patient. The consultant, in turn, seeks to assist the consultee to problem-solve and identify potential solutions.

> This approach in consultation can also serve to motivate the consultee to increase her knowledge base should she become aware of shortcomings. Thus the consultant deals both with a particular problem and the consultee's ability to act on the possible solutions. The more care the consultant takes in assessing and analyzing the data, the more likely the results will be successful. Feedback and evaluation are necessary for both consultee and consultant. (Kohnke, 1978, p. 60)

Teacher

For the consultant, the role of teacher is another "expert" role. Teaching in consultation refers to activities by which the consultant helps his or her client to learn, and emphasizes active learning by the client as a primary goal.

The teaching component of the consultant's role is indirectly related to practice and directly related to the transmission of knowledge on a formal basis. Consulting practice frequently requires continuous training and education within the client system. Seen as a role model by those working within the organizational setting, the consultant can play an effective informal or formal educational role matching teaching skills to the situation. The learning process may involve example and demonstration, may be stimulated through a complex design of objectives and learning content so that others may teach; or the consultant may choose to function as a master teacher.

Researcher

Research or fact-finding is an integral part of the consulting process, whether it be for developing a data base, for diagnosing client problems, or for producing formal research proposals. It is one of the most critical aspects of problem solving, and it often receives the least attention. This function requires development of criteria and guidelines to be used in fact-finding and related investigations, and includes the analysis and synthesis of the facts. Research can be as simple as listening or it may take on the complexity of a formal survey.

ROLE DIFFERENTIATION: COUNSELOR VERSUS CONSULTANT

Counseling and consulting are similar in nature but different by degree. Both are helping relationships that involve significant human interactions. However, counseling never leaves the personal level, while consultation is less concerned with interpersonal processes and more concerned with task achievement.

According to Okun (1985), counseling involves the exploration of feelings and attitudes directed toward helping the individual client understand himself or herself more honestly and openly as a means to resolve personal problems. Consulting, on the other hand, is a planned, purposive, and mutually deliberative process in which the consultant and client set goals and objectives based on perceived need and then develop processes and practices sufficient to meet those needs (Dinkmeyer & Carlson, 1973).

The desirable result of both counseling and consulting is decisive action. However, the goal of counseling, as stressed by Parsons and Meyer (1985), is self-examination and self-analysis. The counselor focuses on positive reinforcement of desirable client behaviors and decisions. For the most part, counseling principles are grounded in mental health concepts and activities. On the other hand, the consultant cares little for the depths of subjective understanding but works instead to help a client achieve preset goals and behavior modifications in the most efficient way possible to accomplish the task. Good results in counseling are the expected behavioral responses. Good results in consulting are the measurable achievements.

Counseling is a skill or role in the field of consultation. Its major function in consultation is to create a climate in which problem solutions may be explored and formulated. Counseling is thus an important skill, and one that the nurse consultant will utilize as needed during consulting encounters.

To further clarify the distinction between counseling and consulting, the following examples are typical of nursing practice in general:

1. The nurse explores attitudes and feelings regarding death with a dying patient. Here the focus is on the client's perception of dying with all its emotional implications. *This is counseling.*
2. The nurse meets with a community group interested in exploring methods of self-care and maintaining wellness. The nurse's methods are health-related and directed toward providing information to individuals that will enable them to establish and maintain good physical and mental health. The nurse guides them to lifestyle changes. *This is consulting.*
3. The nurse meets later with the same group, and the discussion centers on the exploration of individual and group emotions and feelings. Individual opinions and reactions are sought, and the group process involves active participation as group members struggle personally with their decisions. *This is counseling.*
4. The nurse is working with a family regarding follow-up care after hospital discharge. The situation requires mutual setting of very specific goals, with the nurse acting to mobilize the resources of his or her clients and guiding them toward achievement of preset goals in the most desirable and efficient way possible. *This is consulting.*

SUMMARY

Nurse consultants no longer enter a static field in which some of the parts merely need to be rearranged. The settings in which the consultant functions and the roles that he or she assumes are constantly expanding in depth and scope. The professional nurse consultant, acting in an ever-expanding variety of service, administrative, educational, and research settings, becomes more and more aware of his or her functioning level as a consultant, and is thus better able to identify situations that help or hinder his or her performance.

Additionally, effective consulting depends on a clear definition and understanding of the consultant role. A well-known axiom of management theory as stated by Walker (1980), Biddle and Thomas (1979), and Langford (1981) is that the development of an effective organization lies in the division of labor, and that these divisions of labor must be carefully coordinated to prevent disunity. As we have seen with the similar practices of counseling and consulting, the different roles are defined by their activities and functions, and a clear division of labor must be maintained if client goals are to be realized. The differences exist not only in theory but also in the skills and approaches involved.

The consultant who enters the collaborative relationship with a clearly defined role avoids frustration, misunderstanding, role conflict, and failure. The core transaction of any consulting contract is the transfer of expertise from the consultant to the client. This holds true whether the expertise of the consultant is in designing health services, planning and developing, problem solving, team building, or in directing research activities. Whatever the expertise, it is the basis of the consultant's business.

SELECTED REFERENCES

Anders, R. Program consultations by a clinical specialist. *Journal of Nursing Administration,* Nov. 1978, 34–38.

Bell, C., & Nadler, L. *Clients and consultants.* Houston: Gulf Publishing Company, 1985.

Biddle, B., & Thomas, E. *Role theory: Concepts and research.* Huntington, N. Y.: Robert E. Krieger, 1979.

Clark, C., & Shea, C. (Eds.). *Management in nursing.* New York: McGraw-Hill, 1979.

Dinkmeyer, D., & Carlson, J. *Consulting: Facilitating human potential and change processes.* Columbus, Ohio: Chas. E. Merrill, 1973.

Fay, M. Consult a nurse expert. *Nursing Success Today,* 1985, 2(3), 34–36.

Fiedler, F., Chemers, M., & Mahar, L. *Improving leadership effectiveness.* New York: Wiley, 1976.

Kohnke, M. *The case for consultation in nursing.* New York: Wiley, 1978.

Lancaster, J., & Lancaster, W. *The nurse as a change agent.* St Louis: C. V. Mosby, 1982.

Lanford, T. *Managing and being managed: Preparation for professional nursing practice.* Englewood Cliffs, N.J.: Prentice-Hall, 1981.

Lange, F. *An evaluation of the effectiveness of rural health practitioner primary health care clinics in Alabama.* Paper presented at the Fifth Annual Conference of the American Rural Health Association, Lake Tahoe, Nevada, 1983.

Lant, J. *The consultant's kit: Establishing and operating your successful consulting business.* (2nd ed.). Cambridge, Mass.: JLA Publications, 1985.

Lippitt, G., & Lippitt, R. *The consulting process in action.* La Jolla, Calif.: University Associates, 1978.

Margulies, N. Perspectives on the marginality of the consultant's role. In W. Burke (Ed.), *The cutting edge: Current theory and practice in organizational development.* La Jolla, Calif.: University Associates, 1978.

Merry, U., & Allerhand, M. *Developing teams and organizations: A practical handbook for managers and consultants.* Reading, Mass.: Addison-Wesley, 1977.

Okun, B. *Effective helping: Interviewing and counseling techniques* (2nd ed.). Belmont, Calif.: Brooks/Cole, 1985.

Parsons, V., & Meyer, B. *The nurse as counselor*. Reston, Va.: Reston Publishing Company, 1985.

Stanhope, M., & Lancaster, J. *Community health nursing*. St Louis: C. V. Mosby, 1984.

Stevens, B. The use of consultants in nursing service. *Journal of Nursing Administration*. 1978, *8,* 7–15.

Walker, J. *Human resource planning*. New York: McGraw-Hill, 1980.

CHAPTER 3
Exploring Consultation Theory

Theory grows out of the experiences of consultants in practice and then returns as an intellectual structure organizing that practice
                                                    Barbara Stevens, 1979

It should be obvious by now that consultation, as a practice area, covers a wide range of consultant–client relationships, consultant roles, and process structures. The importance of understanding the linkages among these areas cannot be overstated. All our assumptions, beliefs, and personal philosophies are derived out of the mass of data we encounter daily. In order to make sense of this data, we use models or theoretical frameworks. Consultants need guidelines for use in organizing thoughts and making purposeful their behavior in interactions with clients. In short, consultants need to develop a theoretical base from which they can operate in meaningful ways.

Consultation theory and practice constitute an integrity—that is, they are not different things. Effectiveness and success in consulting are based on the ability of the consultant to bridge the gap between theory and practice. Dinkmeyer and Carlson (1973) point out that a consultant must have a theoretical frame of reference that includes a systematic description or analytical theory that provides a set of concepts guiding perception of "what exists," and a diagnostic theory focusing on symptoms or disruptions in the system. Such frameworks play a central role in the nature and quality of consultant performance.

This chapter explores consultation theory by presenting a cross-section of major theories and theorists that helped shape the consulting field as we know it today. More specifically, the chapter deals with the process that explains and clarifies the phenomenon of consultation. As such, this chapter constitutes an attempt both to evaluate the existing theories of consultation and to assess the prospects of prescriptive application.

The proposition that consultation is an important social phenomenon is widespread in the literature of the social sciences, psychology, sociology, human relations, management skills, and organizational development. The concept of consultation is applicable to a wide range of human interactions. Formal references to consultation as a major feature of human exchange relationships are found in discussions of topics ranging all the way from interactions among members of family units to interactions among actors in the international system.

WHAT IS A CONSULTING THEORY?

In effect, a theory is a plan of attack. It is the structure upon which information central to the solution of the problem can be located and placed in perspective, enabling the consultant to develop a sense of the relationship between each of the bits of data. Janice Thibodeau (1983), in her book on nursing models, defines a theory as "a set of interrelated concepts that presents a systematic view of phenomena by specifying relations among variables" (p. 23). Thus, a consulting model provides a roadmap—a way of looking at consultation.

Each of us tends to hold a primary philosophy, based on a number of theories or conceptual frameworks, regarding how best to understand the dynamics of relationships and organizations. It is this mixture and the consultant's right combination of methods and technology that shape a successful consulting endeavor.

Implicit in what has been previously stated is the assumption that existing theories provide a basic understanding of approaches for establishing a consulting relationship. Consultants, in order to evolve a theory of practice, must have knowledge of not only the development of consulting theory but how it is put into practice. Consultation theories generally agree that consulting is a learning process. Differences in theories occur not when the process is put into action but in the discussion of how this learning takes place. Some theorists (later named and discussed in this chapter) argue that it is the nature of the consulting relationship itself that causes client learning to take place—this is the humanistic or person-centered position. Other theorists argue that client learning takes place because the consultant reinforces techniques and facilitates action—this is the behavioristic or task-oriented position. Although these two theoretical positions view the process of change differently, both include a process for change within their theoretical structures.

One prime criterion for a good theory is that it has to be useful. A few of the more useful theories of consulting are summarized in this chapter. Emphasis is given, in the historical overview, to both humanistic and task-oriented theories of consultation as well as the newer eclectic or "choose what you need" approach. In no way is this an exhaustive treatment of the theoretical field of consultation. It is only meant to provide the consultant with a basic introduction to consulting frameworks.

HISTORICAL ROOTS

Historically, consultation has been a field of endeavor so large, complex, and fragmented that integration of its parts has been difficult to achieve. The field has traditionally been comprised of a series of separate camps, such as those of the psychologists, social workers, vocational counselors, marriage counselors, educational consultants, health services consultants, and managerial and business consultants. In fact, according to Lant (1985) there are now over 100 subspecialties in business management alone wherein a consultant might specialize. Each camp has developed its own variety of techniques to use and each camp exists, more or less, in isolation from the others, with little or no benefit from comparison, cross-examination, or mutual stimulation. Hence practitioners have little source of guidance beyond what they have learned from responding to a client's perceived needs or from intervention based on their own subjective preferences and biases.

In reality, many consultants feel that the model of consultation followed by the consultant is not as significant as the consultant's and the client's perceptions of the model's impact. It is important, however, that consultants be familiar with both the theoretical (conceptual) and practical (process) dimensions of consultation. Understanding of the origins of consultation theory is important if consultants are to have the systematic insights needed to guide effective intervention strategies.

THE DEVELOPMENT OF CONSULTATION THEORY

Formal consultation theory first began in the fields of medicine and psychology. For example, according to Shein (1969) the medical or doctor–patient model is traditionally one in which the doctor (consultant) is hired by the patient (client) to discover the source of the problem and to offer solutions without in-depth background data or active assistance from the client. This model is goal-centered and action-oriented; it stresses skills training. The medical model suggests that the best mode of treatment is to train the client directly and systematically in what he or she needs to do to live more effectively.

The major advantage of the medical model, from the client's viewpoint, is the limited time and energy expenditure required of the client. However, disadvantages outweigh any advantage that may exist, in that the entire area of human relations is viewed as irrelevent or untenable, thus resulting in a major communications gap (Stanhope & Lancaster, 1984). As Egan (1975) points out, "the doctor doesn't face just an ulcer in room 436; he faces a human being, perhaps scared and dependent. No doctor can merely assign the patient's humanity to chaplains, aides, or volunteers while he takes care of the body" (pp. 7–8). Neither can the nurse consultant only assess and problem-solve without consideration of the mutually collaborative, "help-ing" relationship wherein the client progresses to a state of independent decision making and acts accordingly.

The principles outlined in the medical model were also true of early mental health consultation in the 1940s and 1950s, which placed emphasis on the "expert" consultant role. In this setting the consultant confers with psychologists and mental health technicians on the treatment aspects of client problems. This third-party approach as a consulting technique is fur-ther discussed in the next section. As more experience was gained with this direct service approach, it was recognized that it would be beneficial to include the client in the problem-solving process. Hence, by the end of the 1950s, a major breakthrough in mental health and business consultation resulted in the client's becoming more active in the consulting process. Carl Rogers (1951) and Gerald Caplan (1959) emerged among the leading repre-sentatives of this approach.

In the 1960s and 1970s business organizations of all kinds—relying on the assumption that consultants had expert knowledge and skills for problem solving—hired consultants to teach both administrative and staff employees in areas of need. Frequently the consultant, in this type of situation, not only did the diagnosis and critical analysis of the problem but also ended up doing the majority of the work toward solving the problem. During the same period of time, educational consultants experienced an ever-increasing demand due to the emphasis on curriculum content and preparation for accreditation enforced by public cries for excellence in educational offerings.

Although many of the varieties of consultant practice mentioned still continue at the present time, there is a rapid movement toward an even more generic purpose of consultation, one in which the consultant facilitates the client's use of his or her own skills and knowledge to resolve difficulties (Shein, 1969). This collaborative approach results in an efficient and effec-tive process whereby clients learn to analyze their own behaviors with the consultant functioning as a catalyst for change. This model is referred to today as process consultation.

The present chapter can only provide a condensed representation of the broad spectrum of the field of consultation, but it is important that the consultant be familiar with a few outstanding leaders in the consulting field.

Gerald Caplan

Gerald Caplan is undoubtedly one of the leading theorists in the field of mental health consultation. He collected his findings, experiences, and re-commendations in his basic text, *Concepts of Mental Health Consultation*

(1959), and has updated his material in several subsequent publications (1964, 1970, 1982). It is interesting to note that much of Caplan's consulting theory was developed from his intense study in mental health consultation with public health nurses as "consultees" in Boston in the 1950s and 1960s. It was during this time that consulting principles took on a primary care focus. His principal developing method was called "crisis consultation." Two separate crises were involved—the crisis in the client and the crisis in the consultee; in this case, the public health nurse (Caplan, 1970).

In his earlier works, Caplan viewed consultation as a three-way relationship of consultant–consultee–client with the consultee being viewed as the professional who works directly with the client. The consultant, in turn, consults with the consultee. Thus, Caplan originally saw consultation as a profession of expert service and collaboration with other professionals. Although these foci are fairly apparent, the nature of Caplan's consulting relationship may need some clarification. According to Caplan, in his explanation of the expert service model, the goal is to assist the consultee to deal more effectively with specific client, program, or organizational problems, with the entire premise being that now the consultee will have the knowledge and skill to deal with similar client problems in the future. Singh and associates (1971) analyzed Caplan's approach to consultation as being client focused but found that his methodology involved seeing or assessing the client only as a means of training the consultee. A clearer explanation of Caplan's three-way consultation concept, as depicted by Singh, is shown in Figure 2. This type of consultation is the basic feature of Caplan's work.

Caplan's concepts are analytic, based upon his clinical experiences, and applied to nonclinical situations in which the consultant interacts effectively with the consultee and the consultee, in turn, becomes more effective in his or her interaction with the client. A good example of this would be the interaction of the nurse consultant with nursing faculty, with the goal being one of improvement of faculty teaching effectiveness with nursing students.

Another example would be the approach of the consultant to community consultation, with the consultant's focus upon working with community

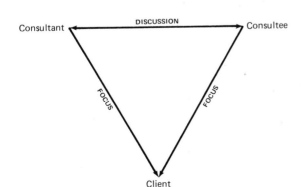

Figure 2. Caplan's concept of the consultant–consultee–client relationship. *(From Singh, R., Tarnover, W., & Chen, R. Community mental health consultation and crisis intervention. Palo Alto: National Press, 1971.)*

agencies, community workers, health administrators, and community leaders interested in building a primary care clinic rather than consulting at the grass-roots level with the personnel that would be working in the clinic itself.

Singh further refers to this relationship between consultant and client as being "egalitarian," that is, as reflecting a belief in the equality of all people. The consultant accomplishes this outcome by enhancing the consultee's understanding of the client. The consultant relates to the consultee on a colleague-like basis; the contract being to examine the problems together. The consultant and consultee share their observations and perspectives, keeping focus on behavior of the client so that they can understand the client better.

Carl Rogers

Like Caplan, Carl Rogers is a humanist in his approach to consultation theory. His orientation to consulting practice is a third-party (consultee–client) approach, as evidenced in his book *Client-Centered Therapy* (1951). He is perhaps best known for his counseling theories of personal therapy (client-centered therapy), a label that describes the fact that consulting approaches revolve around client desires and feelings rather than being directed toward the ideal problem solution. Here the consultant's role as expert and director of the problem-solving process is de-emphasized. Instead, the consultant sets the stage so that clients themselves define their problems, react to them, and take steps toward their solution without specific consultant intervention. Rogerian Theory is phenomenological in that it is concerned with the client's own view of the situation rather than how it actually is (Lefrancois, 1979).

Rogers' works (1942, 1951, 1957, 1961, 1967) emphasize client self-determination rather than the power of the consultant. Still, the skills that Rogers sees as critical to the first stage (entry) of the client–consultant relationship (and actually, to the model in its entirety) are precisely the skills of the consultant process as outlined in this book; that is, communication of respect, genuineness, and accurate empathy, all ways of establishing a truly collaborative consulting relationship.

Kurt Lewin

Kurt Lewin (1951) contributed heavily to the theoretical base of consultation. In pointing out his position, he suggested that anyone involved in helping humans to change has two basic choices. One is to provide direct treatment to the person desiring the change—that is, counseling, advising, and supervising (the humanistic approach). The other choice is, through consultation, to indirectly change the environmental variables of an organization, system, or structure that are causing the problem (the task-oriented approach). Involving people in making decisions about things relevant to their lives is, according to Lewin, an example of indirect treating through changing one element of the environmental structure.

Lewin (1951) originally advanced his force field analysis model as a framework for problem solving and for effecting planned change. Lewin identified pressures or forces in a social system that either strongly supported change or strongly resisted it. His use of the term "force" does not refer to a tangible, physical force but serves as a metaphor for a broad range of influences on the interpersonal functioning of individuals and groups. Lewin's model can be extremely useful to the consultant when it is used to analyze the positive and negative aspects (restraining forces and driving forces) involved in collaborative decision making. The model enables the consultant and client to analyze the various forces and develop strategies for planned change. In effect, Lewin's force field analysis model and his concepts of the consultant as primary force and facilitator for planned change provide the theoretical orientation for the present book, and are further developed in Chapter 7.

Douglas McGregor

Early conceptual work on human motivation in the field of organization development by Douglas McGregor (1960) is another example of utilizing conceptual knowledge to bring about planned change. McGregor's description of the relationships between values and behavior in his book, *The Human Side of Enterprise* (1960), became widely known as theory X and Y— terms that he used to differentiate between two types of assumptions that consultants make about clients. This theory bears repeating because it has applicability not only to consultants but to anyone in a leadership role. The defining characteristics of theory X and Y are briefly summarized in Table 3.

Following identification of the client as having either X or Y character-

TABLE 3. ASSUMPTIONS OF MCGREGOR'S THEORY X AND Y

PEOPLE BY NATURE GENERALLY:	
Theory X	**Theory Y**
1. Do not like to exert themselves and try to work as little as possible	1. Work hard toward objectives to which they are committed
2. Have little ambition or desire for responsibility and prefer to be directed	2. Assume responsibilty
3. Have little capacity for creativity and are incapable of directing their own behavior	3. Are capable of directing their own behavior and want to succeed
4. Avoid making decisions whenever possible and are motivated only at a survival level	4. Are not passive or submissive and prefer making their own decisions
5. Cannot be trusted or depended on	5. If trusted and depended on, will not disappoint
6. Need to be closely supervised and controlled	6. Need support and help

After McGregor, D. The human side of enterprise. *New York: McGraw-Hill, 1960.*

istics, McGregor's aim was then to effectively intervene and foster positive change and goal achievement. There are many versions of these two theories, which are all elaborations or modifications of McGregor's work. One preferred by the present author, since it has specific implications for consultant–client teamwork, was developed by Blake and Mouton (1983). This is shown in Table 4.

McGregor also developed a set of scales that included measurement of high to low ranges of such group characteristics as trust, communication, listening, team objectives, and conflict among group members. One advantage of such a set of scales is that the consultant can point out the problems, ask the group to deal with issues it might recognize as being important prior to the consultation, and initiate discussion of them. The purpose is to provide each member with information about how others perceive the group in comparison with the consultant's perception, and then to provide the group with clues as to how group effectiveness can be improved.

Edger Shein

Edger Shein (1969) followed the work of McGregor in organizational development by giving even more structure to the processes (stages and interventions) involved in the consulting relationship. He is given credit for the term and field of process consultation (also the title of his major work in the consulting field). Shein defines process consultation as "a set of activities on the part of the consultant which help the client to perceive, understand and act upon process events which occur in the client's environment" (p. 9).

According to Shein, the process consultant seeks to give clients "insight" into what is going on around them, and between them and other people. The events to be observed and learned from are primarily the various human actions that occur in normal everyday activities. Of particular relevance in process consultation are the client's own actions and his or her impact on other people. Thus Shein's emphasis, like McGregor's, is to study the human processes that occur in any individual, group, or organization so that they can be structured within a workable framework.

Management Theory

Much of the work behind today's consultation theories was developed, piloted, applied, and synthesized by theorists in the field of industrial management. McGregor's theory X and Y (1960), Likert's management systems (1967), Argyris' organizational development (1970), and Hersey and Blanchard's situational leadership theory (1977) all blend easily with the consultation theory assumptions that client behavior should be self-directed if any permanent behavioral change is to be made.

Management is defined (by Hersey and Blanchard, 1977) as working with and through individuals and groups to accomplish organizational goals. Management theory, by necessity, is directed toward OD (organizational development) and MBO (management by objectives) as the management

**TABLE 4. IMPLICATIONS OF THEORY X AND Y FOR
CONSULTANT–CLIENT TEAMWORK**

IN EFFECTIVE CONSULTING RELATIONSHIPS:	
Theory X	**Theory Y**
1. Authority flows unilaterally from consultant to client	1. Authority flows from formal and informal sources, up, down, and across the consulting relationship
2. Span of control is narrow and there is a need for close consultant supervision of the client	2. Span of control is wide, with supervision of the consultant being general rather than detailed
3. The client is considered an isolated unit, and work is organized primarily in terms of his or her physiological being	3. The client is considered as a social–psychological–physiological being capable of structuring his or her activities
4. Work is routinized, neither creative nor challenging	4. The task is a meaningful whole, providing some creativity and variety, and requiring knowledge, skill and judgment

From Blake, R., & Mouton, J. Consultation (2nd ed.). Reading, Mass.: Addison-Wesley, 1983.

system for controlling and running the organization. Certainly, not many nursing consultants will be involved in large industrial settings, but it is the management concepts of "big business"—motivation, objective-setting, shared responsibility, team development, leadership, and interpersonal skills—that provide the common thread that appears in the definitions of both management and consultation.

Open System Theory

Perhaps the most recent and most popular theory of social change is found in the open systems model. This model views the human being as "an active and proactive agent, purposive in nature and a problem solving organism" (Lippitt & Lippitt, 1975, p. 18), and is regarded by some system theorists as universally applicable to physical and social events and to human relationships in small or large units (Bennis et al., 1976).

In a systems theory, all living systems are open systems—systems in contact with their environment, with input and output across system boundaries. Use of this theory permits examination of the interactions of all actors, both internal and external, who are involved in a consulting setting such as a community.

Thus an open system theory involves a recurring cycle of input, transformation, and output. Both the input and output characteristics of the open system keep the system in constant interaction with the environment, while the transformation process is contained within the system. An effective open system requires a balance among the three stages of the cycle with an input taking into account both environmental demands and the capacity of the transformation cycle, and the transformation process absorbing the flow from the input and moving to the output stage. (Goodstein, 1980 p. 220)

Systems theory presents a problem-solving approach to consultation, and it is oriented to "here and now" analysis as opposed to any future-oriented approach such as the development model. The major drawback to open system theory for the nurse consultant is that it does not provide an operational guide—that is, structural stages and behavioral interventions for consulting with human service systems.

B. F. Skinner and Albert Bandura
Cause-and-effect relationships of high "morale" and personal satisfaction were questioned by B. F. Skinner (1953, 1969) and Albert Bandura (1969) as well as other behavioral modificationists including Scott (1966) and Weiskrantz (1968). These behaviorists or task-oriented theorists hold the belief that a highly structured, clearly outlined task will stimulate self-satisfaction and performance in a causal fashion.

Skinner, for example, contends that automatic reflex responses to stimuli are among emotions that are felt; that feelings are, at best, accompaniments rather than causes of behavior; and that both are common environmental variables. Thus, he supports behavior modification as a concept and feels that a practitioner (consultant or counselor) must have a thorough practical grasp of the basic principles underlying learning, unlearning, and relearning no matter how he or she feels about behavior modification as a technique (Egan, 1975).

Bandura, following Skinner's lead, suggests that self-reports of satisfaction should be treated as simply another class of behavior with no inherent relationship to performance, and that the key to high performance lies in task design.

In consultation the behaviorist theory makes the following two assumptions: (1) that clients have an ultimate goal toward which they are striving and (2) that the ultimate goal can be identified empirically and progress toward it measured (Yuchtman and Seashore, 1967). In fact, this type of orientation to a specific goal is one of the defining characteristics of a consulting relationship in that each stage of the consulting process has behavior and learning that must take place before progress can be made toward goal achievement.

Robert Blake and Jane Mouton
Robert Blake and Jane Mouton, in their widely used text *Consultation*, (1976; 2nd ed., 1983), leave the field of specific theory development and work toward a general theory of consultation and what they term cyclebreaking interventions. They view all behavior—whether that of an individual in solitude, of people within a group, or of people in a larger social setting—as tending to be cyclical in nature. In their words, "a sequence of

behavior repeats its main features, within specific time periods or within specifiable settings" (p. 2). As an example, they cite the alcoholic who starts each day with a drink. The drink is not necessarily at the same time every day and there may be departure from the pattern occasionally. But such deviations are variations on a regular theme.

Cyclical behavior can become so habitual that it is beyond the conscious or "self" control of the person, group, or community whose performance it characterizes. Often this cyclical behavior can be harmful and self-defeating. The consultant's function is to help the person, group, organization, or larger social system identify and break out of damaging kinds of cycles.

Blake and Mouton stress that consultation is a process of breaking cycles, and identify five interventions that the effective consultant employs. These interventions are summarized below.

- *Acceptant.* The intention is to give clients a sense of personal security so that when working with the consultant they will feel free to express personal thoughts without fear of adverse judgments or rejection.
- *Catalytic.* Catalytic intervention assists clients in collecting data and information to reinterpret their perceptions as to how things are.
- *Confrontational.* This intervention challenges clients to examine how the present foundations of thinking, usually value-laden assumptions, may be coloring and distorting the way situations are viewed.
- *Prescriptive.* The consultant tells the clients what to do to rectify a given situation, or does it for them.
- *Theories and principles.* By offering theories pertinent to a client's situation, the consultant helps the client internalize systematic and empirically tested ways of understanding the problem (pp. 4–5).

Some consultant interventions may be "pure" acceptant or "pure" catalytic, and so on; other consultants employ "mixtures" and shift from one kind of intervention to another. According to Blake and Mouton the majority of consultants appear to develop one intervention style and to rely on it, sometimes to an excessive degree.

Since one or another of the five intervention strategies can be used in variety of approaches to consultation, the basic question is: which kind of intervention when? Table 5 shows Blake and Mouton's examples of client situations that call for one or another of these five basic processes.

REFLECTIONS ON THEORY

This summary of the major frameworks for consultation is far from complete. Some authors, such as Barclay (1968), developed conceptual models based exclusively on philosophical theories. Other authors utilized learning theories, organizational theories, theories of leadership and supervision, and educational theories, as well as theories of growth and development and

TABLE 5. USING BLAKE AND MOUTON'S FIVE BASIC INTERVENTION STRATEGIES

Intervention	Key Words	When Indicated
Acceptant	Emotional release	Pent-up feelings are blocking thought and action so that initiatives cannot be taken
Catalytic	Strengthen perception	Poor communication has resulted in pluralistic ignorance that blocks effectiveness
Confrontational	Value clarification	Values, often hidden, are having negative effects
Prescriptive	Giving answers	Clients have thrown up their hands or are on the ropes unable to exercise sufficient initiative to move
Theories and Principles	Insight	Clients are ready to shift to a science-oriented basis for problem solving

From Blake, R., & Mouton, J. Consultation (2nd ed.). Reading, Mass.: Addison-Wesley, 1983.

personality in order to articulate a theoretical base that facilitates the relationship between consultant and client. However, the purpose for the historical review as set forth in this chapter is to emphasize that today two major and sometimes conflicting consulting theories exist—behaviorism and humanism—and that the majority of consultants tend to align themselves with one or the other. Table 6 summarizes the dichotomy that exists between behaviorism and humanism as described by Barclay (1968).

According to Barclay's description, behaviorists are task-motivated. They limit their consulting practice to an objective methodology relying heavily on learning theory with the resultant identification of a problem and devising ways and means to help change client behavior. Behaviorism is generally considered most effective when specific tasks that need to be accomplished are pinpointed. On the other hand, humanism provides a rich background of experience in how to approach clients and build a meaningful relationship. Humanists are relationship-oriented as opposed to task-oriented. The concept of humanism is characterized by such terms as caring, accepting, supporting, empathy, and conscious awareness.

If indeed a dichotomy of theory does exist between behavioral and humanistic theories, then how does a nurse consultant function effectively when confronted with opposite theoretical orientations both of which claim pragmatic effectiveness in the consulting process? It appears that the dilemma of the nurse consultant is to select from a multitude of theoretical structures one or more from which a collaborative relationship with the client can be developed. This textbook proposes an eclectic approach as a solution to the problem.

ECLECTICISM

Increasing disenchantment with the one-sided (behavioristic or humanistic) approaches to consultation theory has led many consultants to favor the use of an alternative model. One of the most popular choices for a consulting model, and the choice of the present author, is eclecticism. An eclectic approach represents the integration of behaviorism and humanism, as illus-

TABLE 6. DIFFERENCES BETWEEN BEHAVIORISM AND HUMANISM

Item	Behaviorism	Humanism
General Orientation	Object-oriented Cultural norms and scientific reality	Subject-oriented Individual understanding and subjective reality
Goals of Counseling	Clarification of individual problems through identification, exploration	Clarification of subjective self-concept and understanding
Methods	Understanding through exploration of environment and scientific knowledge Identification of behavioral deficits Change of behavior through operant conditioning, or social learning theory Removal of maladaptive behavior through de-sensitization, new learning	Understanding of environment and relationship to self Supportive dialogue in exploration of both external and internal environment Changes in self-understanding through insight and clarification
Process Orientation	Change in behavior leads to change in attitudes. Attitudes, feelings, motivation, etc., are concomitants of behavior, and behavior change reinforces reorganization of thinking	Change in attitude, feelings, removal of blocks to self-expression and defensive learning leads to freer expression of ideas and change in behavior
Criteria	Essential reference to external demographic or cultural criteria of assessment. Use of testing information, statistical inference, and scientific research design	Essential reliance on self-report of client and/or evaluation of counselor with some reliance on measurement theory and statistical analysis

From Barclay, J. Counseling and philosophy: A theoretical exposition. *Boston: Houghton-Mifflin, 1968, p. 19. Permission granted by Houghton-Mifflin Company, TSC Division.*

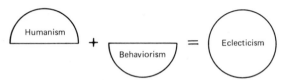

Figure 3. Conceptualization of the development of consultation theory.

trated in Figure 3. The eclectic approach is viable for all phases of the consulting process. It is a synthesis of other theories and yet it is an integrated, consistent and valid system in itself. Eclecticism allows the consultant freedom of choice of both theoretical framework and style of consultation deemed necessary to meet the situational objective.

The word "eclectic" means to select or to choose appropriate sources or systems. The leading proponent of the eclectic viewpoint is Frederick C. Thorne, who in 1945 founded the *Journal of Clinical Psychology*. Thorne contends that a single orientation is limiting and that procedures, techniques, and concepts from many sources should be utilized to best serve the needs of the client seeking help. The true eclectic maintains that there is a consistent philosophy and purpose in the methodology used. From knowledge of perception, development, learning, and personality, the eclectic consultant develops a repertoire of methods and selects the most appropriate for the particular problem and the specific client.

> Eclecticism is a more encompassing system in which all applicable theories, or subsystems, are synergized into a form permitting them to be utilized considerably more effectively than the sum of the parts taken independently. Thus the purpose of consulting would be a synergistic relationship to advance human potential. (Steffire & Grant, 1972, p. 355)

Eclecticism does not negate the need for the consultant to operate in a planned and deliberate manner. On the contrary, the consultant must have some kind of theory in order to organize and understand what he or she sees. The choice of theory, however, remains contingent on the purposeful goals of the consultant process. Fiedler (1967) proposes guidelines to improve leadership effectiveness that are equally applicable for use by the eclectic consultant. He suggests that the behavioristic or so-called "task-motivated" consultants perform more effectively in very favorable or very unfavorable situations, while humanistic "relationship-motivated" consultants perform more effectively in situations intermediate in favorableness. He further classified three kinds of leadership situations:

- *High-control situations* allow the consultant a great deal of control and influence and a predictable environment in which to direct the work of others. This situation usually involves a single client or small group and is best for the task-motivated consultant.

- *Moderate-control situations* present the consultant with mixed problems—either good relations with the group clients but an unstructured task, or the reverse, poor relations with group clients but a structured task. This situation is best for the relationship-motivated consultant.
- *Low-control situations* offer the consultant relatively low control and influence—that is, where the group does not support the consultant and neither the task nor the consultant's position gives the consultant much influence. Stress or high group conflict may also contribute to low control. Some consultants prefer this kind of situation because they enjoy the challenge. Such a situation calls for a high degree of expertise as both a task-motivated and a relationship-motivated consultant (eclecticism) (pp. 10–11).

Thus, eclecticism is flexible enough to use in a wide range of situations and interventions, including individual and group consultation as well as community and organizational development. It is eclectic in that it utilizes several different sources of gain based upon the situational relationship, and multiple social-psychological theories. Choice depends on the knowledge, skills, and judgment of the individual consultant.

Finally, when utilizing an eclectic approach, it is important to keep in mind not only the advantages but also the disadvantages of this methodology. Shertzer and Stone, in their book *Fundamentals of Counseling* (1980), identify some of the criticisms and contributions of eclecticism (Table 7).

TABLE 7. CRITICISMS AND CONTRIBUTIONS OF ECLECTICISM

Some of the more common criticisms of eclectic counseling are the following:
1. The present state of scientific progress does not permit detailing differential treatments for various diagnostic conditions.
2. Achieving facility in a few counseling methods is difficult, let alone achieving skill in a multiplicity of methods.
3. Counselees will be uneasy with changes in methods, and change may only be a counselor's rationalization because the selected method fails.
4. It is doubtful if the counselor can determine the correct or most appropriate method on the basis of immediate client reaction.

The contributions often cited include the following:
1. An attempt at systematization of counseling in itself is valuable and worthwhile.
2. The eclectic approach deals with a wider range of etiologic factors than any single method.
3. Dogma and emotional involvement associated with a single orientation are minimized or reduced.

From Shertzer, B., & Stone, S. Fundamentals of Counseling (3rd ed.). Boston: Houghton-Mifflin, 1980.

THE FUTURE OF CONSULTATION THEORY

Knowledge and the use of theory alone will not guarantee a smooth consulting relationship. For this reason many of the consulting texts presently being published stress procedure, steps, phases, or stages of the consulting process, and behavioral intervention strategies rather than theory itself. For example, besides Blake and Mouton's (1983) previously identified strategies (acceptant, catalytic, confrontational, prescriptive, and theories and principles), Lippitt and Lippitt (1975) explored comparable internal and external consultant intervention strategies as well as identifying 4 sequential stages of consultation as a basis for the consulting process. They labeled these stages as: contact and entry, contract formulation, planning for problem solving, and action-taking. Bell and Nadler (1985) also approach the consulting process from a solely structural viewpoint. Their perception of the consulting stages (structure) include: entry, diagnosis, response, disengagement, and closure. Kinlaw's (1981) model sees the consulting process more from the aspect of activities involved and identifies them as involving, exploring, resolving, and concluding. Thus, the future of consulting appears headed toward a development of consulting practice as a combination of structural stages and intervention strategies as well as a problem-solving, decision-making process. A framework for the consulting process, such as the one presented in Part Three of this book, guides the consultant's activities during all stages of the consulting relationship while providing the freedom and flexibility needed to apply the kinds of specific interventions that will be the most effective for solving specific problems of specific clients. Combined with theoretical eclecticism, the consulting process allows the consultant the freedom to choose theories, sources, or systems that are most appropriate for the time, place, and client situation.

SUMMARY

Faced with the reality of multiple theoretical consulting structures, it is not feasible to speak of a single theory of consultation. Rather, consultation has evolved from a number of theoretical concepts that are not necessarily incompatible. For example, in an eclectic approach, it is possible to use all of the concepts that humanism implies and still make use of the knowledge offered in behaviorism and other approaches.

Accordingly, this chapter deals only with the most important conceptions of consulting as well as the major theories that have been constructed from time to time to explain the phenomenon of consultation. There is, however, a crucial theme that ties all these concepts and theories of consultation together. In every case, consultation is conceptualized as a development process, one through which the consultant and client can reach specific goals or outcomes under conditions of joint collaboration, strategic interaction, and independent decision making. The consultation model in this book can, therefore, be viewed as a process that:

1. Is composed of five progressive independent stages—entry, goal setting, problem solving, decision making, and termination.
2. Utilizes a set of intervention strategies—receiving, informing, facilitating, energizing, and reflecting—to facilitate movement through the consulting process.
3. Employs an eclectic theoretical approach to accomplish the goals of consultation.

Detailed descriptions of these components of the consulting process will be examined in Part II.

SELECTED REFERENCES

Argyris, C. *Management and organizational development.* New York: McGraw-Hill, 1970.

Bandura, A. *Principles of behavior modification.* New York: Holt, Rinehart, and Winston, 1969.

Barclay, J. *Counseling and philosophy: A theoretical exposition.* Boston: Houghton-Mifflin, 1968.

Bell, C., & Nadler, L. *Clients and consultants.* Houston: Gulf Publishing Company, 1985.

Blake, R., & Mouton, J. *Consultation* (2nd ed.). Reading, Mass.: Addison-Wesley, 1983.

Bennis, W., Benne, K., Chin, R., Corey, K. *The planning of change.* New York: Rinehart and Winston, 1976.

Caplan, G. *Concepts of mental health consultation.* Washington, D.C.: U.S. Department of Health, Education and Welfare, 1959; 2nd ed. 1964.

---. *The theory and practice of mental health consultation.* New York: Basic Books, 1970.

---. The modern practice of community mental health. In H. Schulberg & M. Killilea (Eds.), San Francisco: Jossey-Boss, 1982.

Dinkmeyer, D., & Carlson, J. *Consulting: Facilitating human potential and change processes.* Columbus, Ohio: Chas. E. Merrill, 1973.

Egan, G, *The skilled helper.* Monterey, Calif.: Brooks/Cole Publishing Co., 1975.

Fiedler, F. *A theory of leadership effectiveness.* New York: McGraw-Hill, 1967.

Goodstein, L. Consultation to human service organizations. In J. Jones & J. Pfeiffer (Eds.), *The 1980 handbook for group consultants.* San Diego: University Associates, 1980.

Hersey, P., & Blanchard, K. *Management of organizational behavior.* Englewood Cliffs, N.J.: Prentice-Hall, 1977.

Kinlaw, D. *Helping skills for human resource development.* San Diego: University Associates, 1981.

Lant, J. *The consultant's kit: Establishing and operating your successful consulting business* (2nd ed.). Cambridge, Mass.: JLA Publications, 1985.

Lefrancois, G. *Psychology for teaching*. Belmont, Calif.: Wadsworth, 1979.

Lewin, K. *Field theory in social science*. New York: Harper & Row, 1951.

Likert, R. *The human organization*. New York: McGraw-Hill, 1967.

Lippitt, R., & Lippitt, G. *The consultation process in action*. La Jolla, Calif.: University Associates, 1975.

McGregor, D. *The human side of enterprise*. New York: McGraw-Hill, 1960.

Rogers, C. *Counseling and psychotherapy*. Boston: Houghton-Mifflin, 1942.

———. *Client-centered therapy*. Boston: Houghton-Mifflin, 1951.

———. The necessary and sufficient conditions of therapeutic personality change. *Journal of Consulting Psychology*, 1957, *21*, 95–103.

———. *On becoming a person*. Boston: Houghton-Mifflin, 1961.

———. *The therapeutic relationship and its impact*. Madison: University of Wisconsin Press, 1967.

Scott, W. Activation theory and task design. *The American Scholar*, 1966, *35*(2), 275–276.

Shein, E. *Process consultation: Its role in organization development*. Reading, Mass.: Addison-Wesley, 1969.

Shertzer, B., & Stone, S. *Fundamentals of counseling* (3rd ed.). Boston: Houghton-Mifflin, 1980.

Singh, R., Tarnover, W., & Chen, R. *Community mental health consultation and crises intervention*. Palo Alto: National Press, 1971.

Skinner, B. *Science and human behavior*. New York: Macmillan, 1953.

———. *Contingencies of reinforcements: A theoretical analysis*. New York: Appleton-Century-Crofts, 1969.

Stanhope, M., & Lancaster, J. *Community health nursing*. St Louis: C.V. Mosby, 1984.

Steffire, B., & Grant, W. *Theories in counseling*. New York: McGraw-Hill, 1972.

Stevens, B. *Nursing theory: Analysis, application, evaluation*. Boston: Little, Brown, 1979.

Thibodeau, J. *Nursing models: Analysis and evaluation*. Monterey, Calif.: Wadsworth, 1983.

Weiskrantz, L. *Analysis of behavioral change*. New York: Harper & Row, 1968.

Yuchtman, E., & Seashore, S. A systems resource approach to organizational effectiveness. *American Sociological Review*, 1967, *32*(6), 891–903.

PART II

The Consultation Process: Structure, Strategies, and Conceptual Framework

To this point, consultation has been discussed as a viable and multifaceted role for the nurse; settings in which consultation takes place have been explored; the historical roots of consultation have been examined; and consulting theory has been analyzed. It is now time to move into the critical stage: the formulation of a framework for effective consultation—that is, the consulting process itself.

The consulting process should not be a new concept to the professional nurse, since both the consulting process and the nursing process have much in common (their similarities as well as their differences are explored in Chapter 4). But just as the nurse functions within the conceptual framework of the nursing process, the nurse consultant needs a consulting framework. This section fulfills that need.

The consulting process has three distinct yet very much interrelated areas. These areas are defined as structural stages of consultation, intervention strategies for the nurse consultant, and a theoretical framework for nursing consultation. The first chapter in this section, Chapter 4, presents an overview of these three progressive stages of the consulting relationship which interact to build the dynamic process of consultation. Chapters 5 through 7 represent the breakdown and in-depth discussion of each area.

The first area (Chapter 5), structural stages of consultation, is concerned totally with the structural foundation of the consulting process. This foundation consists of a series of five progressive stages or steps. Each stage has a defined beginning, middle, and end, and guides the consultant and client through the consulting process. The five stages comprise (1) entry into the system, (2) goal setting, (3) problem solving, (4) decision making, and (5) termination of the consulting relationship.

Chapter 6 is centered on classifying and defining types of consultant interventions or clusters of intervention strategies that comprise the second area of the consulting process. Intervention strategies—such as receiving, informing, facilitating, energizing, and reflecting—are the special skills that the nurse consultant brings to the consulting relationship. Effective consultation involves practice in making decisions concerning interventions—that is, when to intervene and how. Knowing how and when to intervene is one of the most critical dilemmas that nurse consultants face.

The third major area of the consulting process, that of defining a theoretical framework for nursing consultation, is covered in Chapter 7. An integrating framework that allows the consultant to borrow ideas, techniques, and methodology from other disciplines and integrate them into a personalized practice of consultation, is a must for every consultant. Chapter 7 serves that purpose by bringing consultation theory into a workable framework of practice.

CHAPTER 4

The Consulting Process

When you understand where he is coming from, then what he does makes sense.

Chip Bell and Leonard Nadler, 1985

A necessary ingredient of consultation is that both consultant and client utilize a process that structures certain kinds of skills and knowledge in order to collaborate on an effective level. When the consulting process is working as it should, many dimensions enter the picture. A contract is negotiated, a body of literature arises to give necessary structure to the relationship, ethical issues come into focus, areas of responsibility become differentiated, and the stages of goal achievement are formalized.

The activities, procedures, and processes that the consultant engages in are as individualistic as the needs of the client and the setting demands. Wide differences exist in the nature of the consulting relationship, the skills the consultant brings, the duration of the relationship, the kind of client system, and the methodology used to attain the desired outcomes. It is therefore incumbent upon the consultant to provide meaningful guidelines to the client that clearly state the consultant's definition of the consulting process, the modes that he or she views as most appropriate to the problem situation, and the process stages that both the consultant and client will follow.

Since successful consultation hinges to a great extent on the use and understanding of the entirety of the consulting process, it becomes important to concentrate effort on this area. This chapter as well as Chapters 5 through 7 are designed to explain and clarify the "three-pronged" consulting process that can provide the nurse consultant with an operational design for consultant use (Fig. 4). Each consulting project, whether it lasts for a single session or ten sessions, involves the use of a combination of structure, intervention, and theory on the part of the consultant.

First, in every consultant–client relationship there are five identifiable and sequential structural stages. Skillful consulting is a matter of being competent in the execution of these stages. The stages are progressive in every successful consultation, but it is the behavioral interventions of the nurse consultant that gives them form and the conceptual framework that gives them meaning. It is the interweaving of the three areas—stages, intervention strategies, and theoretical framework—that makes up the totality of the consulting process.

Certainly one cannot say "follow steps one through five of the stages, use the intervention strategies, apply the theoretical framework, and you will invariably be successful in producing changes in the client and in reaching the agreed upon goals." But a working understanding of the consulting process gives the nurse consultant a method that allows him or her to facilitate change. More than anything else, the consultant needs a practical working model that will answer some hard questions such as those defined by Gerald Egan (1975):

- What steps or stages make up the consulting process?
- What skills are needed by the consultant to do it?
- How can these skills be acquired?
- What specifically must the client do in the consulting process?
- What skills does the client need in order to be involved in this process, and how can these skills be acquired?

STRUCTURAL STAGES OF CONSULTATION

The five stages of the consulting process are affected by certain tasks that the participants, the consultant and the client, must accomplish during the course of a successful consultation. These steps, as illustrated in Figure 5, are a logical progression of planned change activities from start to finish, and so it is possible to arrange these stages in small steps that represent that progression.

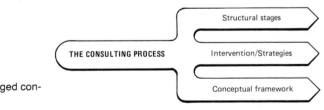

Figure 4. The three-pronged consulting process.

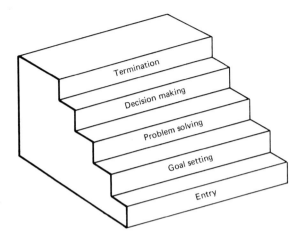

Figure 5. The stages of the consulting process.

Entry
Entry is the first and most difficult part of consultation. It begins with the first contact between consultant and client. This stage can range from a single telephone call to numerous meetings, and may be initiated by either client or consultant. It is a time to ask questions, review capabilities and limits, set time schedules and plan day-to-day operations, and accurately identify the problems.

Throughout the entry stage, both parties explore together the nature of the problem they face and negotiate the specific details and value of the consulting relationship. The primary goals of this first stage are (1) to develop a mutually rewarding consultant–client relationship and (2) to formalize a contract.

Goal Setting
Goal setting is the second stage of the consulting process. Goal setting begins with a clear definition of the problem and specific aim or outcome in mind; at this point, the legitimacy and reality of the desired outcome must be assessed. Ideas are translated into approaches, objectives, tactics, and possible activities that will achieve the worthwhile goal.

Goal setting begins the planning stage. Goal statements articulate direction—that is, they provide a blueprint for the action that follows.

Problem Solving
Problem solving, the third stage, is the creative stage of collaborative consultation. During this continued planning stage, problems are reclarified and possible alternative actions as well as their potential consequences are explored in depth.

Problem solving tells us what is to be done, when it will be done, and how it must be accomplished. In this stage the consultant and client identify resources (both agencies and people) that must be involved in order to move on the plan of action with the best probability of success.

Decision Making

Decision making is the implementation or action stage of the consulting process, and includes the structured activities or interventions employed to correct the problem and reach the goal. In this stage, the client is responsible for taking a necessary course of action. The consultant stands by to help the clients develop their own strategies and tactics as needed for sucessful goal attainment. Figure 6 demonstrates more clearly this process of moving from a confused state of problem identification to a desirable state of action planning.

The decision-making stage is also characterized by a period of testing to determine whether the client is now able to function independently in the new situation. Successful implementation by the client reduces the involvement of the consultant. This gradual separation should lead to a mutually satisfying termination of the working relationship.

Termination

Termination of the relationship is the final step. If all has gone well, termination or closure should bring a feeling of satisfaction to both client and consultant. This stage should be a culmination of careful planning for the disengagement that has been gradually building over the entire relationship.

During the termination stage, the process of evaluation should be evident. Evaluation must now be summarized and shared. If the evaluation shows that objectives have not been met, further work may be indicated. Even if all objectives have been accomplished, both client and consultant may identify the need for periodic follow-up of the situation. Whatever the outcome, the termination should be a formal one. There should be a clearly identified closure meeting for the resolution of all concerns.

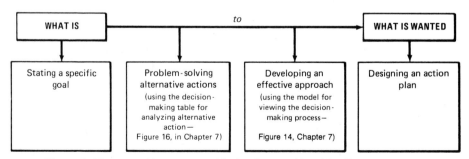

Figure 6. The consulting process: Moving from problem identification to action planning.

INTERVENTION STRATEGIES FOR THE NURSE CONSULTANT

Consultant awareness, knowledge, and expertise in the use of behavioral strategies will facilitate movement through the consulting process. "The linkage between conceptual sophistication, methodological resources, and skilled behavior results from good intervention decisions; decisions by which the client can project, weigh, and choose between action alternatives and activate appropriate behaviors" (Lippitt et al., 1978, p. 38).

Within each stage of the consulting process the consultant utilizes certain learned behaviors (intervention strategies) appropriate to aspects of the situation causing the client's difficulty. For example, during the entry stage, the consultant may perceive the client's reluctance or emotional block relative to a particular item of discussion. An objective and task-oriented approach on the part of the consultant would be completely ineffective in such a case, since the emotional issue would take precedence.

The use of consultant behavior interventions is the second major part of the consulting process. The use of intervention strategies as a vital part of the consulting process is not a new approach. In fact, many authors in the consulting field have built their consulting frameworks around consultant interventions. Robert Blake and Jane Mouton (1983), in their text *Consultation,* provide a classic example of this approach. Blake and Mouton build a total conceptual framework around the consultant's use of five intervention strategies: namely, (1) acceptant, (2) catalytic, (3) confrontational, (4) prescriptive, and (5) theories and principles. Another example can be found in the approach of Lippitt and Lippitt (1977), who combine the consulting stages of contact and entry, contract formulation, planning for problem-solving, action-taking, and continuity with both intervention strategies and eight multiple consultant roles.

This book takes a similar multidimensional approach to the consulting process and identifies five intervention strategies—(1) receiving, (2) informing, (3) facilitating, (4) energizing, and (5) reflecting—as being representative of the behavioral interventions most frequently used by the consultant. These strategies are illustrated as interlocking circles in Figure 7 since, unlike the stages of the consulting process, the five intervention strategies do not necessarily occur in any particular sequence. Rather, these intervention strategies are designed to support and facilitate the change process. Identifying and formulating appropriate behavioral interventions is one of the most fundamental activities of the consultant.

A synopsis of each of the five stages follows. More specific behaviors under each category are further broken down and discussed in Chapter 6.

Receiving

Receiving, as a behavioral mode, frequently occurs during the entry stage of the consulting process. In this stage one of the consultant's biggest chal-

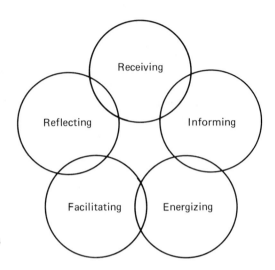

Figure 7. Major intervention strategies
used by the nurse consultant.

lenges is to create a climate in which his or her clients will thrive. Thus, in
the initial process of identifying client concerns and establishing a working
relationship with the client, the consultant nurtures in the client a sense of
personal security. The client, in turn, must feel free to express personal
thoughts without fear of adverse judgments or rejection. In this context, the
consultant is primarily receptive, weighing all the verbal and nonverbal cues
that indicate where the consultant and client may hold congruent, complementary, or conflicting perceptions of the task that they must accomplish
together. Success will not occur in any consulting endeavor without an early
balance of receptivity on the part of the consultant.

Informing

Informing, the next strategy, derives from the more traditional "expert"
role of the consultant. Here the consultant is the expert who, through special knowledge, skill, and professional experience, is engaged to provide a
special service to a client. As an expert, the consultant marshals information
as needed and gives direction to the consulting process until such time as the
client is prepared to accept and act upon a particular approach to his or her
problem. Thereafter, the consultant gradually withdraws from the expert
role to become more of a collaborator and a facilitator.

Informing as a consultant intervention strategy is a necessary and vital
part of any consulting effort. In this mode, the client receives ideas and
information pertaining to the goals that cannot be reached without direct
consultant help. The client retains the final decision-making authority, but
reaches decisions that are clearly influenced by the consultant.

Facilitating

Facilitating as an intervention strategy demands true consultant–client collaboration. The whole atmosphere must be one of joint inquiry and exploration. The consultant strives in a consulting relationship to meet two criteria:

1. The job must be done—that is, the goal should be reached effectively.
2. The client should grow and develop as a result of the consulting relationship.

These two criteria tend to merge since, by definition of the consulting process, clients change to meet their own needs as the goals of problem resolution are approached. Having come to the consultant for help, the clients at some point find the way to help themselves. Often the consultant and client roles are interchangable as they work on a common task and yet, the consultant must always be the "driving force"—the facilitator of the desired outcome.

This intervention strategy of facilitating works to identify those things that impede movement as well as those things that allow for movement. Acting as facilitator, the consultant helps the client to adjust to new perceptions of his or her situation and to take initiative in the problem-solution stage of the consulting process.

Energizing

Energizing is an intervention strategy frequently used when consulting relationships begin to show signs of trouble. Very few consulting relationships run smoothly from entry to termination. Failure to achieve unanimity in a consulting relationship may result in active client resistance.

The process of preventing and handling client resistance to doing the appropriate thing at the appropriate time is largely a matter of understanding the reason for the resistance in the first place. Richard Furr (1979) points out the fact that:

> Resistance is always a motivated behavior on the part of the client, and it makes perfectly good sense to that person to resist. This resistance is often tied to an avoidance of imagined, threatening conditions—a very strong motivation. In such a case it is useful to consider "What could this person be fearing, what is he attempting to avoid by resisting?" (p. 125)

Successful intervention by the consultant should be directed toward minimizing the resistance by stressing the common consultant–client purpose of the relationship. If clients view the consultant's purpose as primarily to get them to take the initiative, they may be inclined to resist. However, if the consultant can relate what is being done to something the client values, the client will be more reluctant to resist. The consultant gains support by providing support.

When energizing strategies take the form of direct confrontation or challenging the client to some form of action, the interaction requires more personal consultant involvement and more expertise in human relationships than any other consultant intervention. The basic process for managing confrontation is influence. The consultant must execute those influence attempts that will move the client toward achieving the client's purpose. In reality, this is consultant manipulation, but it is carried out ethically and purposefully in accordance with the goal of the engagement.

Reflecting

Reflecting is generally an evaluative function. Here the consultant's responsibility is to cognitively map the client's progress or lack of progress throughout the stages of their relationship. Reflecting includes periodic reinforcement and continuous evaluation of change strategies and accomplishments. It is important that clients be made positively aware of their continued advancement toward their ultimate goal.

Reflecting also assists the client's transition from a supportive consultant–client relationship to modes of self-management and levels of achievement that are within the client's reach. Thus, the client has arrived at a decision or a solution and is now able to independently carry out a program for attaining his or her goals. Reflecting, though more pronounced in the final stage of the consulting process, is a continuous function of all consulting relationships from entry to termination.

A THEORETICAL FRAMEWORK FOR THE NURSE CONSULTANT

So far we have considered the physical structure or stages of consultation and the behavioral actions of the consultant. It is the third part of the consulting process, the theoretical framework, that relates the theory presented to actual consulting situations. In consultation this framework is found in the concepts that client change can be planned and solutions can be achieved. During the course of a consulting endeavor, the client makes these key decisions:

1. In the goal-setting stage, clients decide what they want or need a consultant for and thereby indicate a desire to explore their problem.
2. In the problem-solution stage, clients determine how they are going to get what they want.
3. In the decision-making stage, clients decide when they are going to take action.

The consultant enters into the nature of his or her client's dilemma knowing that change is possible through planning and action, and is thus able to guide the client confidently through the shifting balance of direction and action. When clients set goals, they achieve direction; when clients identify their problem, they are poised to resolve it; when they decide that resolution is achievable, they act to realize that achievement.

Additionally, the consultant should always work within the framework of some theoretical model of consultation. A theoretical model provides a roadmap—a way of looking at consultation. It is a representation of reality derived from the successful practice of other consultants. A well-ordered concept of consulting practice will provide a more unified approach to the ordering, selection and rationale for selected actions that have a high ratio of success.

Without a validating theory, the consultant will experience indecision, isolation, communication breakdown, and personal as well as professional failure. A theoretical background will give the consultant the understanding of problem dynamics and interpersonal relationships needed to help the client achieve success beyond his or her own limitations. The models of planned change and decision making designed for this purpose are presented in Chapter 7. The intervening chapters will further detail the sequential stages and the behavioral skills (intervention strategies) of the consulting process, so that we may better understand the context in which consultation, particularly nurse consultation, is effectively applied.

THE CONSULTING PROCESS VERSUS THE NURSING PROCESS

The consulting process utilized by the nurse consultant is synonomous with problem solving and planned change and is compatible with the systematic steps of the nursing process. In the nursing process the steps of assessment—nursing diagnosis, planning, implementation, and evaluation, as presented by Carpenito (1983), Sundeen and associates (1985), and Yura and Walsh (1983)—follow one another sequentially as do the stages of the consulting process. There are close relationships between stages in the consulting process and stages in the nursing process:

1. The entry step of consultation, like the first step of the nursing process, is an assessment stage. Here all the initial data regarding the client's perception of the problem (that is, the physical, social, and emotional environment of the consultant–client relationship), as well as the consultant's perceptions, needs, and conclusions, are assessed and evaluated before the contract with the client is negotiated.
2. The second or goal-setting stage of the consulting process includes the exploration of the client problems for the purpose of establishing client goals. Client goal setting in the consulting process correlates with the goal-setting stage of the nursing process, in that both involve helping the client to set short- as well as long-term goals.
3. Both the goal-setting and problem-solving stages of the consulting process relate to the planning phase of the nursing process, but with

a notable difference in complexity between the two processes at these stages. Although both the goal-setting and problem-solving stages involve collaborative consultant–client planning, the consultant's role provides mainly only guidance and support. Consultation is more an advisory or facilitating activity on the part of the consultant and focuses on stimulating client activities. On the other hand, the planning stage of the nursing process involves more advocacy on the part of the nurse and is usually more directive in nature.

4. The decision-making or client activity stage of the consulting process corresponds well with the implementation phase of the nursing process. Differentiation here is basically the same as between problem solving and planning, in that the activity in consultation is always client activity. In the nursing process, implementation can refer to nursing activity on behalf of the client as well as direct client activity.

5. The fifth and last stage of the consulting process, the termination stage, and the evaluation stage of the nursing process are almost synonymous. Both include evaluation of the attainment or nonattainment of client goals as well as making decisions with the client regarding future needs for the continuation of consultation or nursing care or for the final termination of the relationship.

It is obvious that the consulting process and the nursing process are more alike than different. They both stress collaboration. Certainly, nurses who understand and are skilled in the application of the consulting process will help improve the problem-solving and decision-making skills of their clients. At the same time, the consultant provides the nursing leadership, expertise, and advocacy required by a variety of health situations in many different settings.

SUMMARY

Consultants rely on process. They work in collaboration with their clients through sequential steps, they intervene using appropriate behaviors, and they apply theoretical concepts that facilitate the successful conclusion of the relationship. It is consistent with emerging consultant philosophy that content is less important than process. For example, the consultant is not always functioning in the role of expert or information-giver. Often the consultant is more concerned with the problem of how to go about changing individual client behavior or a situation or system. Thus, the concentration of consultant effort is on change concepts and on mobilizing client strengths.

Furthermore, consultation is the interaction process means through which client goal attainment takes place. The progressive stages of the consulting relationship, the intervention strategies, and the theoretical framework utilized by the consultant to facilitate client movement through the stages, all interact to build the dynamic process of consultation.

SELECTED REFERENCES

Bell, C., & Nadler, L. *Clients and consultants.* Houston: Gulf Publishing Company, 1985.

Blake, R., & Mouton, J. *Consultation* (2nd ed.). Reading, Mass.: Addison-Wesley, 1983.

Carpenito, L. *Nursing diagnosis: Application to clinical practice.* Philidelphia: Lippincott, 1983.

Egan, G. *The skilled helper.* Monterey, Calif.: Brooks/Cole, 1975.

Furr, R. Serving as a messenger: The client-consultant relationship during diagnosis. In C. Bell & L. Nadler (Eds.), *The client–consultant handbook.* Houston: Gulf Publishing Company, 1979.

Lippitt, R., Hooyman, G., & Sashkin, M. *Resource book of planned change.* Ann Arbor: Human Development Association, 1978.

Lippitt, R., & Lippitt, G. Consulting process in action. In J. Jones & J. Pfeiffer (Eds.), *The 1977 annual handbook for group facilitators.* San Diego: University Associates, 1977.

Sundeen, S., Stuart, G., Rankin, E., & Cohen, S. *Nurse–client interaction: Implementing the nursing process.* St Louis: C. V. Mosby, 1985.

Yura, H., & Walsh, H. *Nursing process* (4th ed.). New York: Appleton-Century-Crofts, 1983.

CHAPTER 5

Structural Stages of Consultation

. . . . establish a sound direction with enough flexibility to manage change and produce a constant gain.

Robert Randolph, 1973

All process takes place within a structure that gives it form.

Frances Lange

Consultation is a helping process that takes place in a somewhat distinctive and structured relationship. It is proposed that the basic criterion of such a relationship is predictability. Each consulting project goes through five operational stages:

1. Entry
2. Goal setting
3. Problem solving
4. Decision making, and
5. Termination

Each stage is sequential; if consultants skip one or assume it has been taken care of, they are headed for trouble. Skillful consulting consists of competence in each of these stages. Knowing how to successfully complete the business of each stage is the primary focus of this chapter.

Each of the five stages has consultant and client tasks that must be accomplished before moving to the next stage. Completion of these tasks heralds the reaching of successive goals. It is the client's accomplishment of specified tasks and the indication of his or her willingness to move on that signals a necessary shift in the consultant's role and the move to the next stage.

The following discussion differentiates each of the five structural stages of consultation and includes a brief review of the working tasks (work focuses) that are involved in each of these stages. Included as part of the discussion of each work focus are illustrations of case situations from the author's work experience.

STAGE ONE: ENTRY

Focus of the first stage, entry, is on making initial contact with the client and on settling all the details involved in a consulting endeavor. This first involvement of consultant and client—whether with an individual, group, or community client—begins in one of the following three ways:

1. *The potential client* seeks help because a problem emerges. The problem could be the individual's need for expert information and guidance toward a decision; a group's desire to improve nursing productivity and effectiveness; or even a request from a larger organization such as a hospital, school of nursing, or community seeking the services of a nurse consultant with the knowledge, skills, and judgment the client lacks.
2. *The consultant* makes contact with a client to help correct an identified problem, such as the need for nursing input in a planned community health project or to help a family plan for the future health care of a patient after hospital discharge. Some nurses enter the field of consultation because of their own particular value priorities. Examples might be wanting to provide input in establishing a community nursing clinic, or the desire to participate in policy making of a particular organization through membership in its governing board.
3. *A third party* perceives a need for help in a client system and is aware of the skills and resources that a particular nurse may have as a consultant. This third party could be a friend, family member, fellow worker, unit supervisor, nursing administrator, or just an aquaintance who undertakes to bring the client and consultant together. The referral may be no more than a suggestion to the potential client, or as formal as a three-way meeting. This type of consultation referral happens frequently in the case of governmental agencies or large voluntary organizations such as the American Red Cross or American Heart Association.

Perhaps the best approach to understanding the tasks involved in the entry stage is to take a look at them in their usual order of occurrence.

Marketing

Before the nurse can successfully venture into the consulting field, a systematic approach to planning must answer such questions as: What services should be offered? What will be the target population? How will potential clients be solicited? It is important to understand that marketing one's services is more than merely a prescription for advertising, selling, or promotion. It also encompasses the design, implementation, and control of the type of consulting services being offered.

Eight components are identified by Rubright and MacDonald (1981) as being part of the process of preparing for a consulting career. These components are as follows:

1. *Research.* Carrying out a survey of the consulting field and, more specifically, the opportunities and problems involved with being a nurse consultant. For example, can you travel and be away from home for frequent periods of time? Can you fit consultation demands into your present lifestyle? Are you aggressive enough to run your own business successfully?
2. *The market audit.* Deciding if there is a demand for your expertise and services. Should you function as a full-time or part-time consultant? Should you be an independent consultant or join a consulting group? How will you market yourself?
3. *Setting objectives.* Stating your long-term and short-term goals for your consulting activities. Be specific and include as much detail as possible, as well as a time schedule.
4. *Targeting.* Identifying the population groups (clients) that you feel are best-qualified to help. Gathering statistical data on the needs of the targeted clients. Developing priority lists for contact.
5. *Strategies.* Creating ways and means of marketing yourself and identifying the necessary contacts for the network of resource people that you will need for success.
6. *Special promotional tools.* Arranging for business cards and brochures. Attending workshops, seminars, conventions, and civic group meetings. Participating actively wherever possible. Handing out business cards and contacting your network. In short, being visible and verbal.
7. *Internal adjustment.* Making all of the arrangements needed to be a successful consultant. This includes specifying your time schedule and arranging for office space, insurance coverage, and secretarial help.
8. *Evaluation or recycling.* Reviewing your decisions and consulting arrangements. Have you identified your strengths and weaknesses? Are you happy with your career choice and progress to date?

Although marketing includes a wide range of activities as a part of preparation for consulting, not all of the marketing techniques are used by every consultant. Marketing procedures should be tailored to meet individual consultant needs. Some nurse consultants elect to register with national or even international consultant organizations; others may have brochures designed for survey mailing, business cards and stationary printed, and advertisements placed in professional journals. But no matter what form marketing takes, there is one facet of marketing that should never be overlooked: networking.

Networking, according to Lant (1985), is perhaps the most innovative and successful of the many marketing strategies available to the consultant. Basically, networking is simply making use of potential people resources. These people do not have to be only those who "move in influential circles." The successful consultant lets it be known, to as large a number of business associates and acquaintances as possible, that he or she is available and what type of services are being offered. In terms of money and effort expended, networking is the least expensive marketing technique, and is the quickest method of getting the initial contact needed to build a consulting business.

Another popular method that consultants use to contact potential clients is to advertise in consultant listings in professional journals. The problem with this approach is that the consultant is thrown into competition with many other consultants. This usually results in receiving a number of "form" contact letters of inquiry that are time-consuming to answer and have no guarantee of further acknowledgement. The following is an example of the type of inquiry that a nurse consultant might receive by mail.

> The consultant receives a survey letter of inquiry from a large hospital stating their intention of contracting for the services of a nurse consultant who would work with nursing staff on the writing and implementation of the formalized steps of the nursing process. The letter requests that the consultant send a comprehensive summary of educational background and consulting experiences in the designated area of expertise. If the consultant cannot fulfill this request, or is just not interested in the particular type of service requested, a letter should be sent thanking the potential client for the interest shown but declining a possible contract at this time. If interested, the consultant should respond promptly, showing interest in the project, asking very specific questions regarding the nature of the client's needs, and making sure all of the inquiring letter's specifications are met. This step can be the beginning of a consulting contract. Remember that there will be competition for the position in this type of inquiry and consultants must be prepared to sell themselves (see Chapter 12 for further details of marketing procedures).

The Initial Contact

After finding a client, the consultant's next step should be to determine exactly who the client is and what the client's needs are. Time must be spent, whether by correspondence or in a face-to-face meeting, to explore and define the relationship between consultant and client. The client's wants and needs for services must be detailed, along with the range of services the consultant is willing and able to provide. This period is a time of deciding:

1. What the various parties want from each other.
2. Whether they have the ability and resources to provide what is wanted from the relationship.
3. Whether they are willing to enter into the relationship (Ulschak, 1978).

Like the first phase of the nursing process, entry into consultation is an assessment phase. Here it is important that the consultant assess self-capabilities as well as conduct a careful assessment of the potential client. The objective is to blend knowledge of the client's needs and resources with the consultant's identified needs and capabilities in order to assure production of the data needed for effective problem solving and eventual goal attainment.

The initial interview with the client usually takes place before any consulting contract is signed. On occasion contracts are signed and exchanged by mail, but this could be a risky procedure for either consultant or client, especially if there is no previous knowledge of, or contact with, one another. The initial interview with the client is a time to ask questions, to set limits, to set time schedules and plan day-by-day operations, and to accurately identify the problem. Without the initial interview, there may be neither the time nor the requisite atmosphere to develop an effective collaborative relationship in the future.

The optimal consulting relationship is based on mutual trust and respect. From the standpoint of effective consulting, according to Bell and Nadler (1985), the client–consultant relationship must meet two criteria: (1) the job or project must be done effectively and (2) both consultant and client should grow and develop. Clients accept help more readily from a consultant whose ability they respect. When the relationship is one of acceptance and trust, offers of help are appreciated, listened to, seen as potentially helpful, and often acted upon. Hence the entry stage represents both the initial contact and the beginning of involvement.

Trust in a consulting relationship implies a degree of openness, a spirit of inquiry, and authenticity in consultant–client communication. For example, to evaluate openness there should be an assessment of the responses to such questions as: Is the client willing to set down and explore such things as his or her perception of the reasons for the situation and possible problems that might arise? Does the client appear to have any misconceptions of what the consultant will be able to do? Is the client's mind already made up on a course of action?

If none of the above barriers ensue, the exploratory meeting becomes a major step toward the establishment of a synergistic relationship and the subsequent negotiation of a successful contract. If, on the other hand, it appears that the relationship would be unsuccessful, harmful, or detrimental to either consultant or client, the consulting process should be terminated at this point, or the client referred to another nurse consultant with more specialization in the area of need.

Negotiating a Contract

The initial interview, in addition to being a time for the development of meaningful interpersonal relationships, is also the beginning of negotiations between consultant and client. Negotiating begins with an effort to try to reach an agreement on what particular tasks or series of tasks need to be accomplished, to set a fee, to identify time constraints, to state expectations of one another, and so on (see Chapter 12 for a sample contract of negotiated areas). Virtually all of the duties to be performed, the order in which they will be performed, the person who is responsible for performing them, and the rights and responsibilities that each side has, are decided through a process of negotiating. Negotiations may be completed in a single meeting or may take a number of meetings before mutual agreement is reached.

Contracting is viewed as the formalization of the final decisions made while negotiating. It is essentially a process by which the necessary elements of the desired behaviors are explicitly outlined in a form that is acceptable to both parties. Contracts need not be written, especially in cases where the consultant and client know, or know of, each other and have an unusual degree of mutual trust or have previous experience working together. However, for the consultant entering a complex and unknown working situation, a written document will not only protect the consultant and the client but will help prevent misunderstandings.

Some advantages of a written contract, as outlined by Clark and Shea (1979), are:

1. It provides certainty (given the constraints of language), since there is no need to rely on the memories of the contracting parties, which may become unreliable if there is a dispute.
2. It can specify the binding time deadlines that protect both sides against change without prior notice.
3. It explicitly establishes minimum quality standards for the contracting parties.
4. It specifies the method, form, and time of payment for the contracted goods or services; the procedures for withholding payment; or the penalties in case of nondelivery or delivery of a low-quality product (p. 171).

Hence a contract is, in reality, the development of an action plan. Once consultation has begun, it is always possible and frequently desirable to renegotiate the terms of the contract if situational factors dictate such change (sample formats of both short- and long-form contracts are included in Chapter 12). The signing of a contract usually signals the end of the entry stage. For the purpose of clarity, a summation of the usual tasks involved in the entry stage is given in Figure 8.

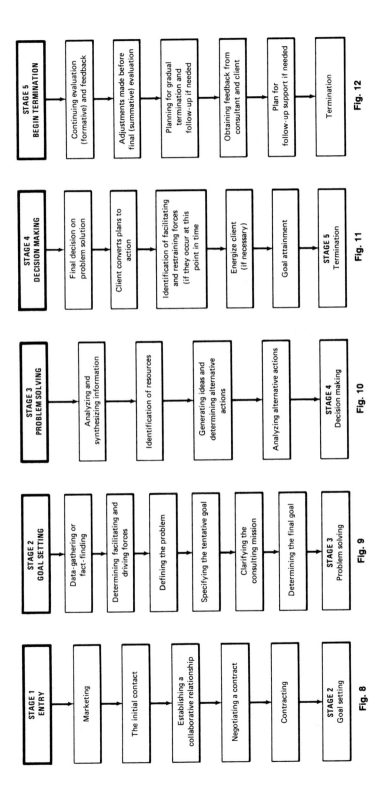

Figures 8 to 12. Major tasks of the entry, goal-setting, problem-solving, decision-making, and termination stages, respectively.

STAGE 1 ENTRY
- Marketing
- The initial contact
- Establishing a collaborative relationship
- Negotiating a contract
- Contracting
- STAGE 2 Goal setting

Fig. 8

STAGE 2 GOAL SETTING
- Data-gathering or fact-finding
- Determining facilitating and driving forces
- Defining the problem
- Specifying the tentative goal
- Clarifying the consulting mission
- Determining the final goal
- STAGE 3 Problem solving

Fig. 9

STAGE 3 PROBLEM SOLVING
- Analyzing and synthesizing information
- Identification of resources
- Generating ideas and determining alternative actions
- Analyzing alternative actions
- STAGE 4 Decision making

Fig. 10

STAGE 4 DECISION MAKING
- Final decision on problem solution
- Client converts plans to action
- Identification of facilitating and restraining forces (if they occur at this point in time)
- Energize client (if necessary)
- Goal attainment
- STAGE 5 Termination

Fig. 11

STAGE 5 BEGIN TERMINATION
- Continuing evaluation (formative) and feedback
- Adjustments made before final (summative) evaluation
- Planning for gradual termination and follow-up if needed
- Obtaining feedback from consultant and client
- Plan for follow-up support if needed
- Termination

Fig. 12

STAGE TWO: GOAL SETTING

Once trust is established and the contract agreed upon, the consultant and client move toward joint exploration of the specific problem. Here the consultant either assists and guides the client in analyzing and understanding the problem, or obtains the needed information to help isolate and identify the problem. Bell (1982) states that the consultant must be confident that consulting activities are congruent with what is needed by the client and consonant with what the consultant can deliver. To achieve congruence and consonance, data pertaining to the problem identification must be gathered, clear goals must be set, and a more comprehensive assessment than that carried out in the entry phase must be made to determine what is appropriate for the situation.

Data Gathering or Fact Finding

Data gathering or fact finding refers to the collecting of information that both consultant and client need in order to understand the presenting problem. No matter what kind of information the consultant seeks, the role is basically that of researcher. It is a very critical area and often the one that receives the least attention in the actual problem-identification process. Data-gathering first requires the development of criteria and guidelines to ensure that all the data needed are collected completely and systematically. It ends when all of the available facts have been analyzed and synthesized by both consultant and client. Data collecting or fact finding can be as simple as listening and compiling facts in a logical format, or as complex as carrying out a formal survey utilizing any number of techniques.

Data gathering for groups is more complicated than individual fact finding only in that it encompasses the interaction of more people. The initial task of working with a group, as with working with an individual, is to observe their interaction and to collect material pertaining to the problem and the goal. Even if the task of the group is very technical—for example, formulating nursing diagnoses and planning nursing care—the interaction of people and viewpoints has to be part of the data collection. The choice of method for gathering data depends on the scope of the study, the time available for the study, the motivation of the client, and the severity of the problem. Block (1981) recounts five ways to collect data.

- *Interview.* Can either be structured (using a set format) or unstructured.
- *Paper-and-pencil questionnaire.* Takes more time to prepare but is good for large numbers of people and is less personal or time-consuming than the interview method.
- *Document analysis.* Looks at records, reports, written communications, and the like. Time-consuming for the consultant.
- *Direct observation.* Can be the best source of consultant data. Obser-

vation of clients in their work settings can take a lot of the consultant's time but is often a worthwhile experience.

- *Your own experience.* Evaluates the data on the client's ability to handle problems and make decisions based on knowledge gained in previous consulting endeavors (pp. 154–155).

When all data are gathered and analyzed, attention is turned to the identification of driving and/or restraining forces that may be present in the individual client (or in the group) and to the additional major tasks of the goal-setting phase yet to be accomplished: that is, specifying tentative goals if needed, clarifying the consulting mission, and determining the final goal.

Specifying the Tentative Goal

A tentative goal statement is only used when there is some uncertainty about what the final goal should be or as to the direction the goal should take. In order to specify even a tentative goal, both consultant and client must still discuss the nature of the problem in as concrete terms as possible. As an example, the discharge-planning nurse consultant must begin a working relationship with the client during early hospitalization if possible. Even in the early stages of any chronic illness, the client must be guided in exploration of future health needs. A client faced with a choice of either an intermediate health-care facility or home health care will require extensive information regarding the services of each before a final decision can be reached and a discharge plan completed.

Early on, during the goal-setting stage, the consultant assists the client to formulate a tentative goal statement whenever the problem is not clearly defined; for clearly defined problems, clarification of the mission and a statement of the final goal may be all that are required. This step is designed to get both consultant and client moving down the path to goal achievement. The tentative goal statement should identify roles of consultant and client as well as indicate possible alternative routes or strategies to goal achievement. Also, the statement should contain a target date for the outcome to be accomplished. A tentative goal statement might read something like:

TENTATIVE GOAL STATEMENT

With the nurse consultant's assistance, and before the end of this month (January), Mr. A. (patient and/or family) needs to make a list of acceptable convalescent-care facilities for continuity of health care following hospitalization.

Clarifying the Consulting Mission

Clarifying the mission involves the reduction of any apprehension by actively involving the client in establishing and determining the type of data required, the manner in which it will be obtained, the persons to be involved, and the target dates for completion. It is apparent in the tentative goal statement cited in the previous section that the nurse consultant and family members would have to talk with or even visit the health agencies under consideration, gather brochures, pictures, and other pertinent materials for the client to review, and consult with the physician before proceeding to the final decision stage.

Determining the Final Goal

Having a precise statement of the tentative goal and having clarified the mission, the determination of the final goal falls easily into place. The final goal statement is the solution to the client's problem. For example, the client's final goal statement might read:

FINAL GOAL STATEMENT

Two weeks before the discharge-planning date, Mr. A. will have decided on the health-care setting where he will receive continued care.

The above examples may appear as an oversimplified explanation of the functions of the goal-setting stage. But in reality all goals, no matter how complicated they may appear, can be stated objectively and in as much detail as needed. Goals are often nothing more than tasks to be accomplished. The major point to remember is that goal statements articulate direction and represent a collaborative relationship of consultant and client based on equal but different contributions.

There is, however, an important difference between the statement of tentative goal and the formulation of objectives that state the most appropriate day-by-day, or meeting-by-meeting, actions that need to be taken in order to facilitate movement toward the final goal. These statements of behavioral objectives, often referred to as subgoals or tasks to be accomplished, are very precise, itemized actions that are realistic and attainable in a short period of time. For example, objectives can be set for each of the meetings (or even for things to do between meetings) and, unlike tentative or final goal statements, may be relevant to action on the part of either the consultant or the client. Again, referring to the discharge-planning example, objectives for an interim time between planned consultant–client encounters might include such consultant objectives as shown in the following example:

CONSULTANT OBJECTIVES: DURING THE NEXT WEEK

1. Obtain literature and specific details on all of the alternate health-care sites.
2. Contact Mr. A.'s family to alert them to the potential discharge plans and arrange for a meeting this week to answer questions and clarify procedures.
3. Attend planned hospital team meeting to discuss Mr. A.'s progress and future needs.
4. Meet with Mr. A. next Monday and review all data gathered this week.

CLIENT OBJECTIVES: DURING THE NEXT WEEK

1. Discuss my future and future health-care needs with my physician, clinical specialist, social worker, nurse consultant, and family.
2. Write down questions that I need to ask to clarify my future.
3. Meet with the nurse consultant next Monday and, with her help, formulate new questions to be answered and the next step to take.

Thus, as this example points out, the movement toward the final goal requires careful selection of a number of subgoals that are very specific. Goal setting depends on what the desired outcomes are and what activities are required to achieve them. However, there are aspects of goal formulation, other than technical considerations, that the consultant needs to keep in mind during the goal-setting stage. These consultant activities drawn from the work of Peter Block (1981) include the need to:

1. Keep simplifying, narrowing, and reducing the list of subgoals and alternate choices so that they focus more and more on the steps the client can logically take. Eliminate unnecessary and unwieldy subgoals.
2. Give a great deal of attention to maintaining a positive relationship with the client. Include the client at every opportunity in deciding how to proceed. Deal with resistance as it arises, even if it does not have impact on the results.
3. Use everyday language. Avoid nursing jargon unless working with a nurse or nurse-group client. Words used by the consultant should facilitate the transfer of information, not hinder it.
4. Treat the client ideas on setting and meeting goals as valid and relevant information. Remember the consultant is a facilitator and not the producer or decision maker.

These four activities affect how the consultant expertise gets utilized, since they involve aspects of technical skill, problem solving, and goal analysis as "givens." "Identifying and formulating alternative paths of action toward change is one of the most creative activities of the change agent" (Lippitt et al., 1978, p. 13).

By now it should be apparent that there is no clearly defined separation between the five stages of the consulting process. Each stage contains elements of all of the other stages, yet each has its own elements of progression. Identifying the problem, setting goals, and designing the action steps and feedback to guide the action involves balancing and blending of all the elements. Figure 9 diagrams the general tasks involved in the goal-setting stage.

STAGE THREE: PROBLEM SOLVING

The third stage in a consulting project, problem solving, involves analyzing and synthesizing information in search of the best solution to the problem. Identification of resources is another important issue. These resources may include areas of present support as well as a survey of potential people, materials, or systems currently attainable that may need to be deployed for problem solving. Resources can be utilized beneficially by both consultant and client. Both translate information or fact-finding insights into ideas about alternative means of action and then into definite interventions for action and change. Thus the resources or the systems that the consultant uses are as important as the support system for the client. The consultant role at this time is to support and encourage the client toward realistic development of how things should be done. It is often helpful to show the client how others have solved similar problems and to demonstrate the results they achieved. For example, an excellent approach for the consultant to use when collaborating with the patient and family to determine the best source of continued health care that will have the greatest probability of success, would be to arrange for family members to visit the health agencies under consideration.

When the client has reached the point of generating ideas, the consultant must facilitate this process. The ideal tool for assisting the client to look at alternate solutions to the problem in order to determine the one that has the highest probability of success, highest value, and lowest risk is the decision table for analyzing alternative actions. An example of this model using discharge planning as an illustration is presented as Figure 17 in Chapter 7 under an in-depth discussion of decision-making theory.

Problem solving is not always as simple and straightforward as selecting a continuing care facility appears to be. Complex situations are not uncommon. They usually involve large consulting projects and large numbers of people. This point is perhaps better exemplified in the following example:

> A consultant is hired to assist a school system and a parent group in designing and implementing a program for the detection and prevention of sexual abuse in elementary school-aged children. The consultant would first determine, clarify, and analyze the clients' reasons and need before attempting to acquaint school and community representatives with all of the possible alternative ways of initiating such a program. These alternatives might include (1) sessions with teachers on how to recognize possible symptoms of abuse, what to do about it, and who to contact; (2) sessions with parents and other interested community members on methods and ways to prevent the child's exposure to potentially dangerous situations, how to open lines of communication with young children, and how to treat children's anxieties and fears about exposure to possible abuse; and (3) sessions with the children to assess their knowledge and explore their feelings of the subject area.

It is easy to imagine all of the complexity and ramifications involved in this type of consulting situation. It would take a great deal of time and client collaboration to determine the probability of success, the value, and the risk to various groups of each of the alternatives. Lippitt and associates (1978) view this exploration of the potential consequences of actions as "anticipatory skill practice," a kind of "let's pretend." The sophistication lies in the projection of "what might actually happen if . . . , " and in this respect the consultant must help the client to develop the action plan in detail—in defining such things as what is to be done, who is to be responsible, and what resources will be needed. Such a project would involve an overall goal and multiple subgoals. It would require taking one step at a time, with problem solving and decision making frequently being concurrent activities.

Like the previous stages of entry and goal setting, the problem-solving stage has certain set tasks that must be accomplished before progression to stage 4. These tasks are represented in Figure 10.

STAGE FOUR: DECISION MAKING

Until this point no direct action on the part of the consultant and client has been initiated to solve the problem. However, with a working relationship established, the client goal well-defined, resources mobilized, and the objectives specified, the consultant and client have collaboratively developed a plan to put into action. This plan tells all parties involved what to do, when and how to do it, who is responsible, and the outcomes expected. The decision for intervention now belongs to the client, the best decision being the alternative foremost on the problem-solving ranking.

In this stage, there is more separation of the consultant and client role than in any previous stage. Such role separation has been frequently compared to those commonly found in a courtroom between a lawyer and a client. The lawyer advises and defends the client, but it is the client who must take action and make the decision to plead guilty or not guilty and who must take the consequences of this decision. Full participation of the client during stage four must be emphasized because the consultant cannot make the decision for the client and has no vested interest in the outcome of the deliberation. An exception to this would be the internal consultant, who would have a vested interest.

Since stage four is an action stage, one of its major elements lies in successfully converting plans into action. This is not always easy for the client to do. Even well-designed plans frequently fail because of the lack of action skills on the part of either consultant or client to carry through the implementation. Implementation involves risk-taking often at crucial times, and it is in this phase that the consultant's role as energizer is all-important. The consultant must provide the client with techniques that will direct client impetus toward desired change. The payoff is in successful action-taking, successful attainment of subgoals, and eventual goal accomplishment.

At this stage of implementation and follow-through, two focuses have been identified. First, it is the function of the consultant to assist in necessary skill development to increase the probability that client action-taking will be successful rather than abortive. Another element of this first focus is the continued importance of support and praise of the client for small successes and the attainment of subgoals on the plan of action. The major motivation for continuing effort comes from frequent experiences of successful movement to the final goal. Introducing skill development activities and initiating "stop sessions" in which to take a look at progress and to review process issues ensures optimal refocusing of energy on the goal to be accomplished.

The second focus is concerned with the mechanisms designed to elicit feedback or progress being made and in involving the appropriate persons in the assessment of this feedback. The continuing assessment of consquences of action is a crucial element of the role during the action-taking stage. Focus should be on the identification of those things that tend to impede movement toward the desired outcome and those things that facilitate such movement. All client decisions made must be analyzed as to their power to inhibit or facilitate goal achievement. The most immediate confronting responsibility for the consultant is that of guiding the client in the selection of the most appropriate action measures for the solution of the problem. It may even, at times, become necessary to revise action and mobilize additional resources whenever blockages and resistance to planned change occur (see Chapter 7 for additional in-depth theory and models for this process of analyzing decisions and unblocking resistance). An effective consultant can stimulate the client to view self-functioning by looking at the kinds of things happening and how results and effective action may be achieved, but the client cannot be forced to change. This distinction is important. One of the guidelines for implementation is to act only after the final decisions are made about what that action should be. The tasks of both consultant and client during the decision-making stage are outlined in Figure 11.

STAGE FIVE: TERMINATION

As a consultation project nears completion, there remains business to be conducted. The ending of a project is viewed as a legitimate stage of the consulting relationship and as another opportunity for consultant and client learning. The goal for the final (termination) stage of the consulting process is to make certain that the client leaves the transaction with an appropriate sense of optimism and direction. It is equally important to be aware of the fact that everything that happens during the consultation influences its conclusion.

The termination stage begins with evaluation. Like all other consulting activities, evaluation is not exclusive to the termination stage. Rather, it is a constant process of monitoring ongoing activities (process or formative evaluation) culminating with the measuring of the final outcomes (outcome or summative evaluation). The purpose of process evaluation is to provide data that will be helpful to both the consultant and client in making future decisions, and to focus early attention on possible defects in the plan so that adjustments can be made before final implementation. The purpose of outcome evaluation is to measure and interpret the degree of success as well as the reason for any deviation from goal attainment during the consulting process and to make a final assessment at the termination of the relationship. Evaluation also serves the purpose of testing the client's ability to be independent of the consultant.

One of the consultant's greatest challenges is to help the client "learn how to learn" and to develop values and skills of self-renewal—that is, to learn how to initiate new cycles of goal-setting, problem-solving, and decision-making behaviors. This challenge means that the consultant must help the client develop and discover internal sources of support for change. Additionally, clients need to develop the skills of being able to evaluate their need for external help, retrieve external sources of help, and use the resources of the system as a core source of energy, stimulation and follow-through on intentions to act (Lippitt et al., 1978). Consultation must have, as part of its design, a plan for follow-up support or provision for a more gradual termination of the consultant's help. Separation should always be a mutually satisfying termination of the working relationship.

It is easy to fall into the trap of either discontinuing the consultation too soon or continuing to work with a client after the real need for services has passed. It helps to remember that the objective is for the clients to be able to do independently the things that they were initially dependent on the consultant to accomplish. This point of client independence is the time for withdrawal and termination. Withdrawal from the consulting relationship can be a special problem for the internal consultant who still continues to work and live in the same environment.

Frequently, final termination is delayed even though the client has attained the predetermined goals. For instance, the client may still retain some feelings of insecurity about being left in complete charge of the future in relation to the problem, and may want to leave future consultation open-ended for further consultation on an as-needed basis. However, no matter what the termination decision, there should be a crisp, clean ending with no misunderstanding or ambiguity. A decision has to be made, whether it is to delay action, redesign and reimplement, or fully terminate. Finally, the consultant needs to recognize and evaluate his or her own successes and failures during the relationship, since this type of introspection will certainly have an impact on the consultant's future. Recognition from the client takes one of two forms; (1) the client's future call or recommendation of the consultant to others, in the case of external consulting; or (2) recognition from colleagues and clients, in the case of internal consulting. A recapitulation of the guidelines for the termination stage is given in Figure 12.

SUMMARY

A few comments relative to the overall assumptions about the consulting process may be useful here in summarizing the consulting relationship as it progresses through the five structural stages from entry to termination.

1. It is necessary to first establish a collaborative relationship before any effective problem solving can be started.
2. It is important to establish a climate and procedures for feedback both between the consultant and client and among the parts of the client system if effective change is to take place.
3. The consultant must continuously assess the readiness and capacity of the client system to change.
4. Because a change situation of this kind is primarily a learning situation, it is incumbent on the consultant to create a series of conditions in which the client system can learn.
5. The consultant must be critical in terms of self-motivations and in terms of types of material presented or help offered. Material should be designed to meet both perceived and real client needs, not only the consultant's perception of those needs.
6. The consultant should be aware at all times that in a healthy change relationship the client can always reject the ideas, the help, and the relationship.
7. In group consulting relationships, it is desirable to create conditions whereby the consultant can withdraw, at least temporarily, so that the group can become independent and grow.
8. It is equally important after an initial change effort that some procedural planning be done for reestablishing the relationship, appraising the interim action, and evaluating the consultant's role.
9. It is desirable for the consultant to be prepared to accept and help develop new role relationships as the client system gets stronger, and moves to a more independent state.
10. The consultant must willingly initiate termination of the consulting relationship when the client is able to do independently that which he or she was initially dependent on the consultant to accomplish.

SELECTED REFERENCES

Bell, C. *Influencing.* San Diego: Distributed by University Associates, 1982.

Bell, C., & Nadler, L. *Clients and consultants.* Houston: Gulf Publishing Company, 1985.

Block, P. *Flawless consulting: A guide to getting your expertise used.* San Diego: Distributed by University Associates, 1981.

Clark, C., & Shea, C. *Management in nursing.* St. Louis: McGraw-Hill, 1979.

Lant, J. *The consultant's kit: Establishing and operating your successful consulting business* (2nd ed.). Cambridge, Mass.: JLA Publications, 1985.

Lippitt, R., Hooyman, G., Sashkin, M., & Kaplin, J. *Resource book for planned change.* Ann Arbor: Human Resource Development, 1978.

Randolf, R. *Planagement.* Austin, Texas: Learning Concepts, 1973.

Rubright, R., & MacDonald, D. *Marketing health and human services.* Rockville, Md.: Aspen Systems Corporation, 1981.

Ulschak, F. Contracting: A process and a tool. In J. Pfeiffer & J. Jones (Eds.), *The 1978 handbook for group facilitators.* La Jolla, Calif.: University Associates, 1978.

Williamson, J. Mutual interaction. A model of nursing practice. *Nursing Outlook,* 1981, *29*(21), 104–109.

CHAPTER 6

Intervention Strategies
for the Nurse Consultant

Consultants offer assistance by intervening—that is, by taking some action to help a client solve his or her problem.

Robert Blake and Jane Mouton, 1983

Each step in the consulting process confronts the consultant and client with a series of intervention decisions and strategies. This will be true whether one is an internal or external consultant. Effective consultation thus requires a certain selectivity and flexibility of response in the form of intervention strategies (Lippitt & Lippitt, 1975). This chapter explains some of the intervention strategies most commonly used by the nurse consultant.

Intervention strategies are defined here as special consultant skills that are needed to support the client's change efforts. Intervention occurs whenever a consultant does something to or for a client that may initiate a planned change sequence toward client goal attainment. Each intervention calls for behavior on the part of the consultant that will, in turn, release forces in the client that facilitate collaboration and a mutually satisfying working relationship between consultant and client.

Intervention strategies are not sequential in the same sense that the stages of consulting are. However, some stategies are more likely to occur in the early stages of consultation, and others come into play more frequently in the middle or late stages. Intervention strategies are most likely to occur in the order presented in this chapter, although any of the strategies can also occur at other times in the consulting process.

A consultant does much the same thing whether working with one person, a group, or a community organization. There is a consistent use of self to assist the client in many different ways. More than most nursing roles, the nurse consultant role relies heavily on the motivations, relational style, and personal dynamics of the individual performing the role. The multidynamics of the consulting relationship are difficult to analyze.

> This is because consultation does not leave a clearly defined, well bounded, and carefully delineated niche in a system. It is a more amorphous function and much more dependent on personality differences than any other role. It places great demand on the consultant as the instrument of influence and impact on a system. (Rhodes, 1974, p. 290)

The consultant has an almost limitless range of behavioral and human sciences upon which to draw. However, these sciences do tend to cluster, and desirable consultant behaviors can be grouped or categorized into a more simplified model of five major intervention strategies:

1. Receiving,
2. Informing,
3. Facilitating,
4. Energizing, and
5. Reflecting

Each of these intervention strategies is characterized by distinct emotional approaches, cognitive styles, and manners of behaving toward others. At different stages of the consulting process, the client demonstrates different attitudes, different coping styles or expectations toward the work and goal, as well as varying levels of commitment. Any successful intervention by the consultant, across a time span, will include multiple modes of intervention. Individual consultant behavior has to be shaped and developed just as the stages of the consulting process are structured.

The five intervention strategies may manifest themselves in many ways in a client relationship depending on what the focal issue seems to be. For example, during the entry stage the consultant may ascertain a reluctance on the part of the client to enter into a frank discussion of the task to be accomplished. In this case, an approach of being objective and task-oriented would be completely ineffective or might even result in alienation of the client, since the emotional issue would take precedence. Thus, only strategies designed to create a climate of acceptance and open communication—receiving strategies—would promote productive interaction between consultant and client at this point. Generally, receiving interventions are used more frequently early in the developing consulting relationship; but even during other stages of the consulting process, if emotional tensions again become evident, the consultant should turn away from task-centered activities in favor of reestablishing an emotional climate conducive to optimal consultant–client function.

Similarly, the other four intervention strategies are utilized more in certain stages than in others, but are not mutually exclusive. Each intervention category envelops a number of other similar behavioral interventions that are closely interrelated. These are included as subcategory strategies. For example, the behavioral interventions included as part of the receiving category are those of accepting, awareness, empathy, encouraging, genuineness, and listening—all having the single characteristic of helping to build the type of consultant–client relationship most conducive to successful consultation.

The intervention strategies included in this chapter are comprehensive, yet certainly do not comprise all of the possible behavioral interventions used by consultants. All consultants develop their own individualized techniques and strategies for handling the aspects of situations that are presently causing the client difficulty.

RECEIVING

The problem faced by both consultant and client, especially when they first attempt to enter into a working relationship, is a complex one. The problem revolves around the attachment of a new person (the consultant) to an existing individual, group, or community system (the client). Examples include assignment of a nurse consultant to an existing nursing staff, introduction of a nurse consultant to a community health board, and the one-to-one contact between the nurse consultant and a hospital or clinic patient. In each of these cases, the consultant is presumably the expert, the one hired to solve the problem; at the same time, being new, the consultant is relatively unpredictable, just as the situation itself is unpredictable to the consultant.

Hence, one of the consultant's biggest challenges is to create the type of climate where the client will be motivated to achieve the desired goal. In this initial process of identifying client concerns and building a synergistic working relationship, the consultant is the receptor or receiver of all the verbal and nonverbal cues and the emotionally charged experiences that might block productive functioning.

> Being completely objective would imply being emotionless and much else that is not within the scope of any human being. Yet the ability to take an objective view of the situation, or of oneself, or of both, is an essential first step toward tackling many self-defeating cycles. (Blake & Mouton, 1983, p. 14)

The use of receptor interventions by the consultant has the effect of helping the client to think through a problem situation in a manner that relieves the blocking aspects and ensures the client a sense of personal ownership in resolving problems. If, for example, the client is a director of nursing functioning under conditions of emotional stress by virtue of having been "forced into" a consulting relationship by the hospital administrator, the consulting relationship would probably be ineffective until such time as the tension has been dissipated. However, the consultant could facilitate the relationship through expertise in receptor strategies such as:

1. Helping the client think through the situation.
2. Intervening more actively by creating conditions under which the client can problem-solve in a planned constructive manner.

The major gain to the client from consultant use of receptor strategies is that once emotional undercurrents are expressed at the surface level and discharged—at least temporarily—then it may be possible for the client to orient thinking about the problem along more objective lines.

Early successful consultant use of receptor strategies is crucial to the total effectiveness of the consulting process. If the consultant does not possess these skills, then the consultant is going to be ineffective since, as a general rule, progress in consultation can take place only to the degree that the preceding phase has been successful. According to Egan (1975) the ways in which receptor strategies are expressed may change somewhat as the consultant moves deeper into the consulting process, but the need for these skills never disappears.

Receiving can also be described as a social-influence process. If the consultant is going to influence the decision making of the client, then the consultant must establish a positive basis for this influence. Through all the stages of the consulting process, if the consultant is genuinely sincere and receptive to the client, the client comes to see the consultant not only as an expert but as a person who can help provide direction in solving existing problems. In this sense, the skillful consultant establishes good rapport with the client in stage 1 (entry) and engages the client in ongoing constructive collaboration during the entire consulting process.

When working with groups, the basic purpose of receiving as a strategy is to make the group sensitive to its own internal processes and to generate, on the part of the group, some interest in analyzing these processes. In the early stages of a project, some time at the end of each session should be devoted to specific dimensions: that is, how involved the group felt in the process; how clear communications were; how well member resources were used; and so on. Time spent promoting mutual respect and understanding in the early stages will greatly facilitate the later stages of the process.

Used in the context just discussed, it becomes apparent that "receiving" is more or less a catchall term for a number of other interrelated consultant behaviors such as accepting, awareness, empathy, encouraging, genuineness, and listening. These consultant behaviors are important enough to warrant summarization.

Accepting

Accepting is the ability of the consultant to give the client a sense of security, so that when working with the consultant, the client will feel free to express personal thoughts without fear of adverse judgments or rejection (Blake & Mouton, 1983). Acceptance does not depend on the consultant's approval of the client's actions or vice versa. Rather, it implies consultant understanding of what the client believes or feels, and allows the client the freedom to think and feel without fear of criticism or blame from the consultant.

Awareness

Awareness is the development of consultant sensitivity to both the external and internal climate of the consulting process. The consulting process of being with another person is impossible without awareness. As simple as awareness is, it is amazing how often consultant and client fail to attend to one another. Lack of awareness in human relations is quite common and can be disastrous in a consulting relationship. For this reason alone, awareness is recognized as a major receptor skill for the consultant.

Empathy

Empathy is the ability of the consultant to enter into the life of a client—that is, to see the client as he or she is and to accurately perceive the client's current feelings (Kalish, 1973). Empathy is not sympathy. A sympathetic consultant loses identity and actually assumes the identity of the client. The empathic consultant offers support and understanding and still maintains his or her own identity. The best way for the consultant to show empathy is to work to understand the client in terms of feelings, experience, and behavior. The communication of accurate empathy is the real work of stage one; it is work that requires consultant skill and patience.

Encouraging

Encouraging is the ability of the consultant to stimulate active client participation in the consulting process. Here the consultant reinforces positive client contributions and directs the attention of the client to developing more fully the talents already present. This arrangement becomes increasingly more important when working with groups, since the consultant must attempt to involve each group member in the democratic process of planned change.

Genuineness

Genuineness refers to the consultant's ability to reflect his or her self in an honest manner during the relationship with the client. This means that the consultant should be without front or facade, and be open about the feelings and attitudes that are present and of influence during the consulting relationship. Being genuine in one's relationship with another is a way of showing respect.

Listening

Being an evaluative listener is crucial to an effective consulting process. All consultation starts with listening. First the consultant listens and captures mentally, or in written form, the essence of the problem presented. Next, the consultant listens for cause and effect, for discrepancies between stories, for dissonance or turbulence, and for other symptoms of stress. Listening must also be attuned to giving heed to signs of a healthy relationship, such as respect, confidence, trust, and openness. Ferguson (1968) views the consultant as a radar device that picks up blips and cues from listening and then differentiates normal, acceptable cues from those that deserve further investigation and treatment.

The above-mentioned interventions are a small sample of what could be included as examples of receiving strategies. Such consultant responses as attending, consistency, observing, reinforcing, respecting, and understanding are equally important. The point is that unresolved interpersonal conflicts, the lack of mutual support and personal satisfaction, and the failure of the consultant to listen and understand what the client is saying are all issues that, when ignored, frequently immobilize the consulting process. The social-influencing relationship between consultant and client is a delicate balance and the consultant must judge, on the basis of knowledge and experience, what the appropriate receiving strategies need to be for the consulting relationship to function with any degree of effectiveness.

INFORMING

The consultant is employed by a client who assumes that the consultant possesses sufficient expertise and information in the problem area to enable the client to produce answers. Information that the client needs is imparted to the client until such time as the client, now in collaboration with the consultant, can make a sound diagnosis of the problem, problem-solve it, and design a plan of corrective action.

Identifying and supplying information needed is analogous to the approach of the nurse who, after listening to the patient's comments, makes a diagnosis and institutes interventions to correct the problem. Steele (1979) made an even more interesting comparison by contrasting the expert consultant with the classic British detective:

> Clearly, one of the major activities of the detective is an extensive search for clues and evidence as to what has occurred in a specific situation. . . . The detective's reason for wanting evidence may be described as falling into two categories: one need is to gather clues to help him understand what has occurred in a given criminal situation, and a second need concerns using that understanding to search out more adequate evidence to prove to others what has occurred and make a case which can stand up in court. Both of these seem to be of vital importance to the consultant as well. A consultant who focuses attention on active intervention in an organization must be continually seeking to understand the data with which

he comes into contact. And it is of great value to collect and organize these data in such a way as to provide clear, straightforward evidence to the client system supporting the points which he will use trying to bring about change in the system. (p. 130)

For the consultant, it can be personally gratifying to be perceived by others as someone who really "knows what is going on" or what should be done in a given situation. An additional bonus is that the client is often quite happy to have someone take over the responsibility. This shift in responsibility may have some benefits, such as making it more likely that the consultant will be listened to, but it also has some costs. One cost is the potential price in terms of increased dependence of the client on the consultant, a dependence that may keep the client from developing the strengths and competencies needed to solve the problem. A second cost, less often considered, is that a reliance on the consultant as the exclusive expert may often lead to inadequate decisions and certainly ones that are not mutually developed or synergistic to both consultant and client. It is important to realize that although the consultant may gather a large portion of the data by actually doing things and by acting in the system itself, it is always the collaboration with the client that is the vital link to the success of the consulting process. The consultant should never engage in action for action's sake, particularly since this always seems to detract attention from the client and aborts any attempt to form a collaborative relationship.

Argyris (1970) emphasizes the fact that engaging in some behavior simply because it fits the client's expectations or value system may end up limiting the usefulness of the consultant to the client. For example, the oncology clinical nurse specialist hired as a consultant to assist staff to set up policies and protocols for a highly specialized hospital unit, such as a radiation or chemotherapy treatment area, takes it upon himself or herself to do all the research, program design, and protocol writing, with the rationale of saving an already overworked staff time and effort. Consequently, the staff feels left out of the whole experience and ends up resenting and even resisting following the guidelines as developed by the consultant.

Supplying the needed information and functioning in the role of expert is a necessary and vitally important consultant role, and yet it is one of the most difficult for the consultant to handle without succumbing to the tendency to take over. The ideal context for intervening is to do so only when the client seeks ideas and information pertaining to the accomplishment of tasks that he or she cannot reach without direct consultant help and then always leaving the final decision-making authority to the client. In this way, decisions themselves are only facilitated and influenced by the consultant's input as to "how" to achieve the goal.

Informing, like the first category of receiving, is not a self-limiting behavior. There are a number of subcategory bahaviors (related interventions) such as observing, defining, validating, and involving that are just as important to successful consulting. These terms are self-explanatory and are so much a part of informing that they need no separate explanation.

FACILITATING

As an intervention strategy, facilitating focuses on those behaviors or knowledge deficits that tend to impede movement toward the desired outcome and those behaviors or knowledge that facilitate such movement. Clients are likely to encounter problems accomplishing subgoals or tasks and the consultant will be confronted by the responsibility of guiding the client through the exploration of alternative possibilities and the generating of criteria for selection of the most appropriate action in terms of these criteria.

Even after goals are firmly established, a client may be hampered by not being able to understand a situation or not seeing it clearly enough to take needed actions. Although emotions may be involved, the actual cause is frequently lack of data and know-how for accomplishing the specific task. In intervention, the consultant as facilitator enters the situation with the intention of increasing the rate at which a process is occurring. The consultant's ability to stimulate the client to move ahead is the real meaning of facilitation.

The consultant employs a number of approaches to gain cooperation from the client. As an example, Parker (1975) offers a consultant's description of a facilitator intervention used in a hospital infection control program.

> Mentally, rapid judgments and adjustments have to be made as different problems and grades of staff are encountered in the course of a day. It is important to be available to anyone, as far as possible, at any time, which of course means constant reassessment of priorities, or ability to delegate and keep routines to an essential minimum. Both flexibility and resilience are needed. (p. 53)

The facilitating task for the consultant involves helping to clarify issues, options, and strategies for achieving goals, and helping to clarify factors that might be important to the decision-making activities of the client. In working with groups, the consultant serves to link people or groups that need to be brought together in order to achieve the goals of the system—both substantive achievement goals and affiliative human relations goals.

Facilitating starts in the earliest stages of the consulting process and continues throughout the project. The term itself is so broad and all-encompassing that it has few specific comparable strategy components. Such terms as gate-keeping, goal-tending, and team-building are all involved with facilitating, but their function is basically the same. Only one strategy, advocating, is important enough as a substrategy for consideration here.

Advocating

Advocating refers to consultant endeavors to influence the client. Bell and Nadler (1985) emphasize the fact that in consultation there are two quite different types of advocacy:

1. Positional or content advocacy, whereby the consultant tries to influence the client to choose particular goals or to accept particular values.
2. Methodological advocacy, whereby the consultant tries to influence the client to become active as a problem solver, being careful not to become an advocate for any particular solution.

These types of consultant advocacy differ somewhat from what the nurse is used to as a nurse advocate, which is generally defined as one who intervenes on behalf of the client. Perhaps an even better term than advocacy, in the case of the consultant, would be influencing.

ENERGIZING

Values direct both consultant and client behaviors. They may have different cultural, socioeconomic, or spiritual backgrounds that may create a temporary (or even permanent) block to the orderly progression of the consulting relationship. Failure to achieve unanimity will result in disruption, resistance, or even antagonism on the part of the client. If such a block occurs, intervention by the consultant is usually directed toward confronting the client with the realities of the problem and attempting to motivate the client to explore both the factors actually operating within the situation and the possible consequences involved. It is the consultant's way of handling the problem situation and energizing the client that results in the client's being able to successfully break out of self-defeating cycles of behavior and get on with goal attainment. Energizing, as an intervention strategy, is viewed in this context as the force moving the client when such a force is needed.

Blake and Mouton (1983) refer to energizing strategies as confrontational interventions necessary whenever an individual or intergroup relationship becomes "set" or "frozen" in ways that make needed cooperation difficult. This type of situation, which usually occurs during the decision-making stage of the consulting process, forces the consultant to take a stand that challenges the client to some degree of action. One of the most basic issues of energizing or confrontational consultation is the power/authority ratio in the consultant–client relationship. For example, if the consultant enters a consulting situation with a poorly defined problem area and a poor delineation of the consultant role, the consultant is unlikely to be listened to no matter how valid the interventions may be. This division of power/authority teeters on a delicate balance. On the one hand, if the consultant power/authority base is equal to that of the client and shared, then a successful basis of intervention may be established. On the other hand, if the consultant's power/authority base is significantly stronger than the client's, interventions are likely to be responded to as though they were expert directions and taken at a level of absoluteness that they in fact do not deserve. Bell (1982) compared role power to electricity and personal power to having the right appliance. The consultant is better off seeking the right appliance than pursuing greater voltage.

Energizing may also be the intensifying of an action. In the case where a "total block" between consultant and client occurs, the consultant may, instead of requesting, elect to "demand" by issuing an ultimatum or a threat to dissolve the consulting relationship. The following is an example of blocking that requires such confrontation as an energizing consultant intervention:

> A community group intent on building a nursing clinic in their neighborhood have already held a number of meetings trying to come to some decision on a building site. All of the previous meetings ended in disagreements and arguments mainly because of the strong personal involvements of some of the group members preferring one clinical site over another. No one will give in. Things now appear at an impasse, frustration is at a maximum, and the entire project is in danger of collapsing. The nurse consultant has already tried all of the problem-solving and unblocking approaches possible. The consultant now decides that it is time to confront the group and advise them that he or she will dissolve the relationship in one week if they do not make a decision.

This tactic is a drastic intervention strategy and not one to be used in every (or even in many) consulting relationships. When necessary, however, this type of confrontation has the effect of moving the client to examine the status of the situation. By experimentally intensifying an action or an emotion, a person may be able more accurately to identify its underlying characteristics and restraining properties.

Energizing intervention strategies require more personal involvement and more experience in human relations theory than other consultant interventions. Weisbord (1978) made an interesting observation regarding "unblocking" interventions when he stated that "expressing the resistance does not melt it: it makes it real" (p. 19). Thus, when a client is in crisis, the external threat of failure is a dependable incentive when used effectively.

REFLECTING

The ongoing sequences of consultant intervention strategies generally take place at successive moments of time and the role of the consultant in reflecting is descriptive of the decision-making and closure or termination stages of the consulting process. By this time, opposition no longer exists, and in the case of a group or community, the client in effect has joined forces. This assimilation process, or fusion of the consultant and client, is a natural and normal process in a successful consulting endeavor whereby the goal is now attainable and there is agreed-upon joint action.

In this sense, reflecting as an intervention strategy is associated with feelings of accomplishment and success when the client sees the continued advancement of his or her ultimate goal. Patten (1979) compared the optimal consulting process to an overview of the developmental model whereby the individual or group tends to develop from a sustenance level focused on gratification through concrete and tangible incentives, through a level of self satisfaction, and on to a generativity level. At the generativity level the focus of the need shifts from the development of the self to the expression of the client's unique capacities and highest potentials toward goal achievement.

The consultant responsibility as a reflector is, more or less, to cognitively map the client's growth, achievements, and future potential. The client now makes the final decision and is thus able to shift to a systematic methodology of behaviors that include:

1. Knowledge of the specific steps of problem solving and the skills to be able to use it effectively
2. Ability to use a structured model for analyzing alternative decisions according to their high or low probability of success, value, and risk
3. Ability to avoid adverse reactions by being able to explore and analyze forces that may be hindering or restraining constructive activities
4. Capability of ensuring that actions decided on are carried out

Another consideration during the termination stage is whether or not some continued reflection—or in this case monitoring by the consultant—is desirable in the future. Periodic reinforcement and providing for continuous evaluation of change strategies may be needed. The consultant frequently needs to modify plans and review change strategies if and when they fall short of expectations. For example, the community contracting for a nurse consultant's help to build a nursing clinic will probably need the maintenance services of the consultant on an intermittent (as-needed) or continuous basis until the project is self-sustaining.

SUMMARY

The idea of "getting other people to do what you want them to do" raises uncomfortable feelings for many consultants. Yet consultants are expected to have the ability to encourage others to change certain aspects of their behavior. Inexperienced consultants in particular encounter difficulty in "explaining" the character of their consultant behavior mostly because the modes of intervention they use are a "feel as you go along" approach. The behavioral interventions presented in this chapter are designed to furnish the consultant with techniques to help clients make decisions about whether, when, and how to change their behavior. These intervention strategies in interaction with the consulting stages and the consultant's conceptual framework form the basis for the entire consulting process.

The fundamental task of the nurse consultant involves intervening wherever and whenever needed to help the client sift through data and formulate possible alternative actions for the solution of the problem, make decisions, and act to achieve a goal. Consultation may also mean assisting the client to identify feelings that are influencing behavior and inhibiting task completion with the rationale that these feelings may be channeled into constructive behaviors or they may be attenuated. In any case, consultation is consultant support of the client and does involve the intervention of the consultant in a variety of intervention strategies.

The consultant intervention strategies of receiving, informing, facilitating, energizing, and reflecting are broad categorizations. The use of these strategies by the consultant is designed to expedite client decision making. Although there are no guaranteed ways to change client behavior, it is possible through the use of appropriate intervention strategies to increase the likelihood of effecting planned change.

SELECTED REFERENCES

Argyris, C. *Intervention theory and method.* Reading, Mass.: Addison-Wesley, 1970.

Bell, C. *Influencing.* San Diego: Distributed by University Associates, 1982.

Bell, C., & Nadler, L. *Clients and consultants.* Houston: Gulf Publishing Company, 1985.

Blake, R., & Mouton, J. *Consultation.* (2nd ed.). Reading, Mass.: Addison-Wesley, 1983.

Egan, G. *The skilled helper.* Monterey, Calif.: Brooks/Cole, 1975.

Ferguson, C. Concerning the nature of human systems and the consultant's role. *Journal of Applied Behavioral Science,* 1968, *4*(2), 179–193.

Kalish, B. What is empathy? *American Journal of Nursing,* 1973, *73*(9), 1548–1552.

Lippitt, R., & Lippitt, G. *The consultation process in action.* La Jolla, Calif.: University Associates, 1975.

Parker, M. Clinical nurse consultant in infection control. *Nursing Mirror,* 1975, 49–53.

Patten, T. The behavioral science roots of organizational development: An integrated perspective. In J. Jones & J. Pfeiffer (Eds.), *The 1979 annual handbook for group facilitators.* La Jolla, Calif.: University Associates, 1979.

Rhodes, W. Principles and practices of consultation. *Professional Psychology,* 1974, *8*, 286–292.

Steele, F. Consultants and detectives. In C. Bell & L. Nadler (Eds.), *Clients and consultants.* Houston: Gulf Publishing Company, 1979, pp. 119–128.

Weisbord, M. Input versus output-focused organizations: Notes on a contingency theory of practice. In W. Burke (Ed.), *The cutting edge.* La Jolla, Calif.: University Associates, 1978.

CHAPTER 7

A Theoretical Framework
for Nursing Consultation

Frameworks are essentially roadmaps to enable those traveling on the path to effectiveness to anticipate special vistas along the way. Frameworks also allow us to notice time without being a victim of time. They provide a structure which facilitates the release of insight and creativity.

Chip Bell, 1982

Models can be powerful aids in pointing to areas our minds should explore and in surfacing the gaps in our thinking which should be filled.

Chip Bell, 1982

Although the presentation of existing theories of consultation in Chapter 3 is consistent with and important to the understanding of the concepts underlying all consulting activities, effective consultation lies in the selection of a framework that works with a high probability of success. The consultant must have a focus of reference for interpreting the vast amount of data communicated in a consulting session, and the consultant must be able to design strategies that will help the client interpret that data and deal with the situation.

This chapter supplies such a framework for the consultant to use to help bridge the gap between theory and practice. Based on a workable approach built from two major, interlocking theories, planned change and decision making, the two models presented in this chapter provide the consultant with the means to communicate meaningfully to the client all important aspects of the consulting process. The models allow both consultant and client to get an overall picture of the results of individual transactions by providing a simple, but very useful, means of organizing data and detailing relationships between the data elements. Furthermore, the models are designed to record and structure what actually is happening and provide reliable working tools for understanding the nature of the problem, for making decisions about the course of action, and for managing the new direction once it has been defined.

The author will first discuss a theoretical framework for planned change and decision making, and will then take a look at the development of a workable structure for nursing consultation.

THEORIES OF PLANNED CHANGE AND DECISION MAKING

Chapter 3 discussed the historical roots of consultation and described a number of theories applicable to the consulting process. It is now time to focus on the presentation of the theoretical structure for nursing consultation.

To be effective in the role of consultant, the nurse needs to do more than just understand and predict behavior. It is necessary to develop skills in directing, changing, and controlling behavior. Thus, the nurse consultant must be, in essence, an applied behavioral scientist.

Learning to apply behavioral science is much like learning anything else—that is, it must be done by practice, by doing what you are attempting to learn. If the theoretical framework presented in this book is going to have an impact on the reader's knowledge, then the reader must be willing to "try it" and to "use it" consistently in order to feel at ease and for help in becoming a more effective consultant. Hersey and Blanchard (1977) state that "it is this unfreezing that we have to go through if we want to learn" (p. 12).

A WORKABLE THEORY

Planned change is defined by Bennis and associates (1976) as "a conscious, deliberate and collaborative effort to improve operations of human systems . . . through the utilization of valid knowledge" (p. 4). As a process, it centers around a structure aimed at helping the client to become more adaptable and more open to change through the client's use of internal and external resources rather than relying on consultant help to produce such a change.

The primary need for the consultant is to develop a method for managing change that capitalizes on and utilizes the client's own potential for problem solving, decision making, and creativity. It has been the author's experience that the adaptation of Kurt Lewin's work on force field analysis provides one of the simplest and easiest methods for the nurse consultant to understand and use. Thus, it is Lewin's work that serves as the theoretical structure for this book's consulting framework.

Kurt Lewin in particular is credited with the origin of classical change theory, and developed such parameters when he created what is now recognized almost universally as the basic outline of the change process. His work (1951) on the theory of force field analysis still provides the basic theoretical structure for many of the planned-change and decision-making theories as we know them today. Lewin describes three steps in the change process: (1) unfreezing, (2) moving to a new level, and (3) refreezing. In consulting, unfreezing is characterized by the client's recognition of the need for a change resulting in openly seeking help from a consultant. Secondly, the move to some new state or level is brought about by altering and manipulating the problem situation in such a way that the client can clearly define the problem, project goals for the change effort, plan actions that support the change, and implement change in order to achieve the desired goal. The third step, refreezing, is the stage in the change cycle in which the newly acquired behavior is integrated into the client's personality. Table 8 illustrates these concepts by showing them in relationship to the structural stages of consultation and by specifying the parameters for each.

The second part of Lewin's theory on planned change centers on the development of a model of process analysis that allows the consultant to assist the client to define and view both the driving (facilitating) and restraining (inhibiting) forces involved in any given situation. Lewin's model (Fig. 13) offers a methodology for identifying pressures or forces in a social system that either strongly support change and decision making or strongly resist it, thereby inhibiting change behaviors.

The concept of field plays a central role in Lewin's system. Initially it was taken to mean the environment, but subsequent development of the force field theory has also included cognitive meaning. Thus, a field is defined by Lefrancois (1982) as not only, or even primarily, the physical environment, but also the beliefs, feelings, goals, and alternatives of an individual or group. Hence, the model is useful as a means of interpreting interpersonal functions within individual, small group, or community interactions as well as tasks to be accomplished.

The conceptual framework in this book proposes the use of an adaptation of Lewin's model (Fig. 14), as one of two workable models for nurse consultants to use whenever they are involved with the client in the problem-solving, goal-setting, or decision-making stages of the consulting process. This model, combined with a second—a model for analyzing alternative actions—serves as the basis for defining nursing consultation.

The First Model

When using the model for viewing and analyzing driving and restraining forces that facilitate and impede movement toward client goals (Fig. 14) the following procedural steps apply:

TABLE 8. SOME ASPECTS OF CONSULTATION AND MANAGEMENT OF PLANNED CHANGE

Consulting Stages	Lewin's Stages	Parameters
Stage 1: Entry	Unfreezing: Creating motivation to change	1. Client dissatisfaction with the present system 2. Consultant promotes the client's willingness to change 3. Consultant motivates the client in the direction of the hoped-for change 4. Rapport is established between the consultant and the client 5. Consultant and client identify forces in support of the change and those forces that fail to support or are against the change
Stages 2, 3, and 4: Goal Setting, Problem Solving, and Decision Making	Changing: Developing new responses based on new information, making decisions, and acting to promote the desired change	1. Consultant provides client with information needed and with the theoretical knowledge of how to use it 2. Consultant promotes client change in values and attitudes where needed 3. Consultant and client collaborate in diagnostic formulation and reformulation of issues 4. Client analyzes alternative problem-solving solutions and decisions 5. Client takes action and moves to new level of behavior
Stage 5: Termination	Refreezing: Stabilizing and integrating the changes	1. Consultant supports and reinforces client's new behavior 2. Client integrates new responses into personality 3. Client integrates new responses into significant ongoing relationships through reconfirmation

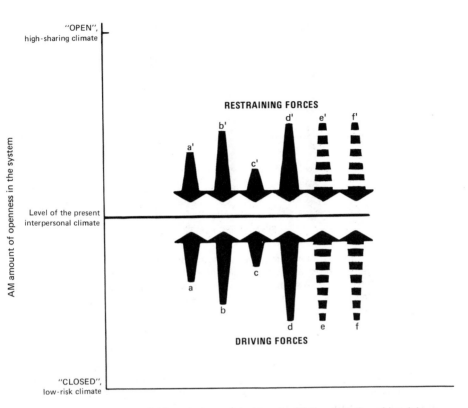

Figure 13. The force-field analysis model of Lewin. (*This adaptation of Lewin's work is reproduced with permission of Pfeiffer, J.W., & Jones J.E. (Eds.). The 1973 annual handbook for group facilitators. San Diego: University Associates, 1973.*)

1. Specify the change desired (the goal, subgoal, or task to be accomplished) using concrete, measurable terms.
2. List all the factors that may influence the situation.
3. Sort the list into the two categories of driving and restraining forces.
4. Array the two lists on the diagram and label them for reference.

With the use of this model, the process of decision analysis is simplified for the client, because he or she can objectively interpret the helping forces as well as the particular problem situation. Only when clients know what they are faced with, and realize the implications of the identified strengths and weaknesses, can they move to correct their position. The changes necessary for goal achievement are accomplished by strengthening the driving forces, weakening the restraining forces, or both. The model enables the consultant and client to analyze the forces one by one, and to identify the individual strategies for dealing with each.

The advantage of this model is its simplicity. The concepts of Lewin's

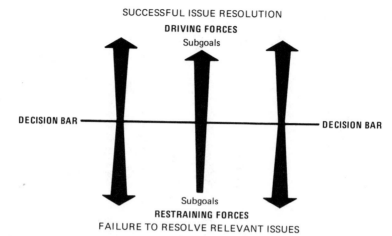

Figure 14. A model for viewing and analyzing driving and restraining forces. *(From Lange, F. The design and development of a rural nurse practitioner primary health care clinic: A study of the decision-making process with emphasis on the role of the nurse consultant. Unpublished doctoral dissertation, The University of Alabama at Birmingham, 1979.)*

freezing, moving, and unfreezing (change process), combined with the application of his force field analysis, provide both a theoretical framework and a model that nurse consultants can use whenever they are involved in analyzing and interpreting client situations. An example of their use by the nurse consultant is given in the next section.

Application Example. The unfreezing process started when a staff nursing group, trying to implement primary nursing care in an orthopedic hospital unit, decided that they did not know exactly how to do it and requested the services of a nurse consultant to help them. Once the group, with the assistance of the consultant, accepted the overall concepts of primary nursing, the consultant's next move was to ask the group to think about the driving and restraining forces that were present in the situation. In thinking about the driving forces that were pushing for the change they wanted, the nurses were quick to name the enthusiasm and commitment of the nursing director, the unit head nurse, the unit RNs, some nursing students, and the fact that it should markedly improve patient care and patient–nurse communication.

In thinking about restraining forces, the nurses began to mention one thing after another. First of all, the nurses stated that they had never had a good relationship with the chief of orthopedic surgery; and that some residents and interns as well as the day shift nursing supervisor were opposing the reorganization of the unit, pointing out that it would probably require a larger nursing staff to implement and that since things were going well there was no sense in "upsetting the apple cart." Using a variation of the model for viewing the decision-making process (Fig. 15) suggests the relationship

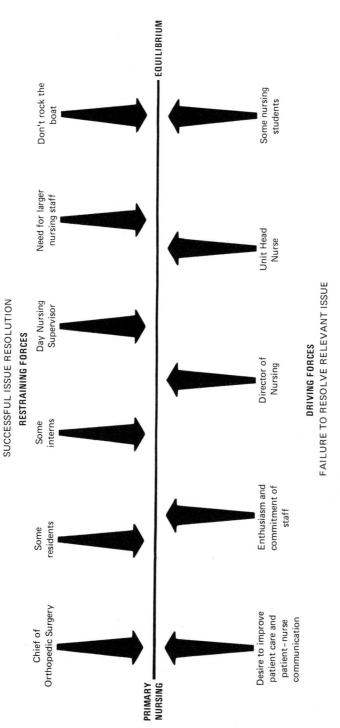

Figure 15. Viewing and analyzing the driving and restraining forces.

between driving and restraining forces in this change situation. As can be seen, the driving forces and restraining forces were fairly well balanced in number although probably not in power. The consultant was able to point out the need to formulate and present a workable plan to the administration that would demonstrate (1) the advantages of primary nursing care to both patients and staff, (2) a step-by-step smooth transition from functional to primary nursing care, and (3) the satisfactory utilization of staff so that no additional nursing personnel would be needed.

The consulting process was again brought into action to help the group move toward a course of action that might help decrease the strength of the restraining forces and increase the strength of the facilitating forces. Following an analysis of these forces, they now selected activities, prioritized by the group, that would help attain the goal. Such activities might include:

1. A gradual implementation of primary nursing in unit X in blocks of 10 beds at a time (biweekly).
2. A weekly evaluation of progress and reidentification of the facilitating and restraining forces that may be affecting progress.
3. An orientation meeting (to be conducted by the consultant) for auxiliary staff of other related units to explain the program and gain their cooperation.

Finally, following implementation and evaluation of their progress, the staff continued to integrate their newly aquired behavior by moving to help other hospital units implement primary care (refreezing).

This situation demonstrates how planned change theory meets the consultant's need for an organized structure from which to function. It is obviously much easier to convert a resisting force to a driving or helping force when that force can be objectively identified. For example, if a client who opposes a change can discover that it offers significant benefits, and that he or she may have overestimated its negative impacts, the client may change from an opponent to a supporter. This change of client attitude or behavior has the double effect of eliminating a force from the restraining side of the field and adding one to the driving side.

Another more specific example would be in an educational setting, where the consultant may find strong resistance from one or more of the nursing faculty when trying to implement an integrated curriculum from one that has been theoretically and clinically separated. Resistance will persist until the benefits of the new curriculum can be clarified as being beneficial to student learning without the sacrifice of learning experiences valued by the faculty. An additional benefit of the new curriculum may be in the form of less actual time involvement in clinical activities by faculty themselves, resulting in their becoming supporters of the changes instead of resisters. In effective consultation, this phenomenon of change from resister to supporter will occur over and over again.

The Second Model: A Decision-Making Model for Analyzing Alternative Actions

Whether working with an individual, group, or community, the consultant essentially utilizes a series of decisions within a structure of planned change. The core of consultation lies in the ability of the consultant to direct, guide, and support clients in their decision making. It is therefore important that decision errors be kept to a minimum. Successful consultation can only be accomplished through the knowledge, practice, and continued use of a formalized process of mutual decision making.

For example, Bales (1960), Lange (1979), Mitchell (1980), Read and colleagues (1977), and Simon (1971) have all stated that we make decisions under three conditions: certainty, risk, and uncertainty. Decisions made with certainty require that the outcome of each alternative be known—that is, that the client knows what the results and penalties of a particular action or lack of action will be. Decisions made under risk are those in which the client can estimate the chances of an outcome but has no way of knowing for sure what might happen. Decisions made under uncertainty have relatively unknown outcomes with many uncontrolled, unknown, or chance factors.

Decision making is a problem-solving process and, as such, has similar steps to follow. They include:

1. Deciding that a client problem or need exists
2. Identifying all possible actions that could be taken
3. Determining the probability of success, the value, and the risk of each action
4. Choosing an action based on high probability of success, high value, and low risk (the ideal solution)
5. Implementing the action
6. Evaluating the action

It is an additional safeguard to use a visual decision-making table. This step is a fairly simple procedure. The second model involved in this book's theoretical framework, which can be used for all decision-making situations, is shown in Figure 16. This model, known as a decision-making model for analyzing alternative actions, allows the consultant to plot with the client not only all possible actions that can be used to solve a problem but also to consider the probabilities of success, the expected values to be attained, and the risks involved in any single decision. A more specific example of its use is demonstrated in Figure 17. Note that there is only one ideal solution that meets the criteria of high probability of success, high value, and low risk. In reality, there may be more than one ideal solution and other decision criteria such as cost, family stress, and so on, may be used. On the other hand, none of the solutions may reach the ideal, and the client may have to choose one with only medium probability of success, value, or risk. The model as shown will satisfy most require-

---

Make a statement of the problem:

List all the possible decisions or actions the patient could take to solve the problem:	Determine the probability of success for each possible action:	Determine the value to the patient of each possible action:	Determine the risk to the patient of each possible action:
1.	High	High	High
2.	Medium	Medium	Medium
3.	Low	Low	Low
etc.			

Choose the action to be taken (the ideal solution is one with a high probability of success, a high value, and a low risk).

Figure 16. A decision model for analyzing alternative actions. *(Adapted from Mitchell, P. Concepts basic to nursing. New York: McGraw-Hill, 1980.)*

ments for effective decision making, but there should not be any hesitation about adding additional categories when indicated.

Decision making is a skill that can be learned, taught, and improved upon. Use of a decision-making table makes it a clearly articulated and structured process. Furthermore, the possibility of error can be minimized when consultants structure their own and their clients' decision making theoretically. In time the decision-making process will be internalized, becoming part of everyday thinking.

Perhaps the most important aspect of the use of the two models presented here lies in the ability of the consultant to put it all together, use it as a meaningful whole, and transfer this knowledge and ability to conceptualize to the client. An illustration of the overall sequence of events in a consulting project is given in Figure 18.

Statement of the problem: Need to decide the best place for follow-up care for Mrs. Brown (stroke patient) upon hospital discharge.

Possible Decisions or Actions	Probability of Success	Value to the Client	Risk to the Client
1. Convalescent hospital	High	Low	Low
2. Nursing home	Medium	Low	Medium
3. Home health care service	High	High	Low
4. Home with visits to hospital clinic	Low	Medium	High

Choose the action to be taken: Home health care service meets the ideal criteria of high probability of success, high value to the patient, and low risk.

Figure 17. Analyzing alternative actions to promote planned change.

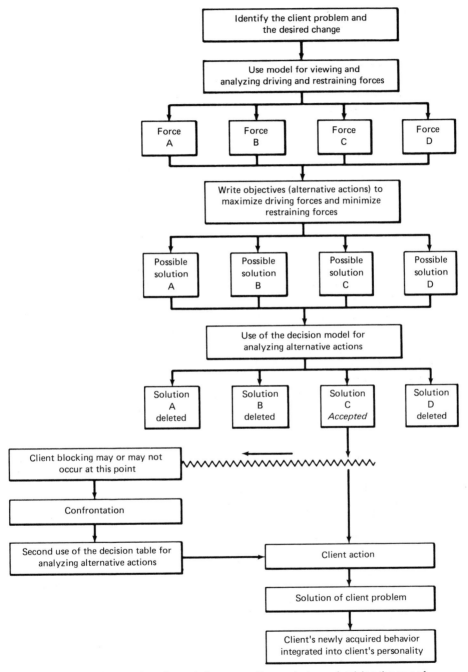

Figure 18. Sequencing of events in a consulting project, emphasizing the use of the models for promoting planned change.

A DISCUSSION OF FRAMEWORK

Thus far in this chapter, the theoretical frameworks of planned change and decision making have been discussed and models have been presented for viewing and analyzing driving and restraining forces and for analyzing alternative actions for more effective client decision making. However, even the use of these models, as presented in Figures 14 and 16, does not guarantee success. Clients at times still act impulsively and make risky choices that turn out far from desirable. When the client fails and turns again to the consultant for help, it can create a dilemma for both parties. No one likes to be told that they were wrong and that is why they failed. Certainly recrimination or even sympathy is not the answer. Only an objective approach with clearly defined boundaries can formulate a clear understanding of what happened and provide answers.

The process of analysis is simplified once the issue is identified for the client as a workable unit. The two models presented in this chapter are intended to facilitate the client's change process, but they are certainly not the only ways to promote change. They are, however, the methods that the author has found to be most effective in the majority of nurse consultant–client encounters. They work well in all individual, group, or community settings, or in any situation where multiple factors (people, issues, facts, beliefs, choices, and so on) are involved. In some consulting projects, the consultant may not need to use both of the proposed models. For example, many consultants have discovered that the decision table for analyzing alternative actions (Fig. 16) is applicable to just about all consulting endeavors while the model for viewing and analyzing driving and restraining forces (Fig. 14) works best in group and community settings.

One benefit of working with these models is that their use helps build the client's understanding of the change process so that the knowledge gained can be meaningfully transferred to similar future situations. This internalization of theory by clients is perhaps best demonstrated by considering a common consulting situation.

Application Example. A director of nursing, at the request of a hospital nursing staff, has hired a nurse consultant to assist the staff to implement the nursing process at a higher theoretical level than that presently in use. The entire process sounded exciting to the staff and the consultant was welcomed with open arms. The consultant planned a series of formal lectures and informal group working sessions for staff that included semiweekly meetings for the next two months (a total of 32 hours of class work). The implementation of the planned change—a complete revision of nursing care plans—also meant home study and multiple written assignments.

After the first three weeks, staff enthusiasm began to dwindle, and people began to miss meetings, pleading mostly lack of time or illness. The consultant realized that she was losing her audience, and identified her

problem as the fact that her groundwork for consultation had been ineffective. She recognized that she had not involved all of the staff in her theoretical orientation to the total consulting process, with the result that some staff
members now felt that they were not an integral part of the relationship. At
this point, the consultant took time to reestablish the consulting relationship, and began to involve the staff with an analysis of the driving and
restraining forces that were now involved in the situation. Only when the
staff was able to freely express and list these forces were they able to reach a
clear perspective and begin to identify possible actions to overcome or neu-
tralize the negative factors. The project then moved rapidly as the consultant assisted the staff to analyze each of the potential solutions as to its
probability of success, its value, and its risk. Thus, consultant use of a
conceptual framework had the effect of breaking the damaging cycles of
behavior that had been present in the situation.

Theory should be an intergral part of the entire consulting process. The
theory part of consultation is twofold: one is the consultant's use of theory
to guide intervention strategies from entry to termination of the relationship, and the second involves the consultant's teaching theory to clients so
that they in turn can use such systematic insights to phase out their own
self-defeating cycles.

SUMMARY

To the extent that consultation involves theory as well as practice, consultants are likely to need skills beyond those of diagnostitians and facilitators.
At the moment, there are few models describing these skills, and little
understanding of how consultants can be trained to acquire them. Based on
theories of planned change and decision making this chapter contains two
such models: one that allows identification, interpretation, analysis, and
evaluation of the driving or restraining forces that may be involved in the
decision-making process, and one designed to promote effective decision
making by structuring all alternatives according to probability of success,
value to the client, and client risk.

One thing the consultant must always keep in mind is the fact that client
problems may or may not be well defined when the consultant enters into
the relationship. It may be difficult to isolate the problem and its related
components, especially when the client does not possess the knowledge and
experience to objectively analyze the situation without consultant help. If
sufficient time is not taken, at this point, to build an effective helping
relationship, the consultant and client can operate at cross-purposes. Conflict can result. Preventing this type of confusion is the major purpose or
argument for the use of models. A model provides not only a tool for

analysis but also promotes feelings of personal growth, awareness, and the building of confidence in both consultant and client.

The use of the theoretical framework as presented in this chapter enables the consultant to avoid two major problems common to consulting endeavors: (1) it guards against subjectivity on the part of the consultant by focusing on a micro-level analysis of the decision-making process, preventing over-generalization; and (2) it conveys credibility to the whole consulting relationship by providing a codified procedure for the transition from data to theory and thence to reality.

The major gain in the use of a theoretical framework is that it provides not only the consultant but the client with a cognitive map for effective problem solving in the future.

SELECTED REFERENCES

Bales, R. *Interaction process analysis.* Cambridge, Mass.: Addison-Wesley, 1960.

Bell, C. *Influencing.* San Diego: University Associates, 1982.

Bennis, W., Benne, K., Chin, R., & Corey, K. *The planning of change.* New York: Holt, Rinehart & Winston, 1976.

Hersey, P., & Blanchard, K. *Management of organizational behavior.* Englewood Cliffs, N.J.: Prentice-Hall, 1977.

Lange, F. *The design and development of a rural nurse practitioner primary health care clinic: A study of the decision-making process with emphasis on the role of the nurse consultant.* Unpublished doctoral dissertation, The Unversity of Alabama at Birmingham, 1979.

Lefrancois, G. *Psychcology for teaching* (2nd ed.). Belmont, Calif.: Wadsworth, 1982.

Lewin, K. *Field theory in social science.* New York: Harper & Row, 1951.

Mitchell, P. *Concepts basic to nursing.* New York: McGraw-Hill, 1980.

Read, D.; Simon, S.; & Goodman, L. *Health education: The search for values.* Englewood Cliffs, N.J.: Prentice-Hall, 1977.

Simon, S. The search for values. *Edvance,* 1971, *1*(3), 1.

PART III

Nursing Consultation in Action: From Concepts to Reality

"I was hired not to do but to think" is a common axiom heard in reference to consulting. Effective consultation is "getting other people to do what you want them to do." This goal often raises uncomfortable feelings for the consultant and others involved. Yet clients must change certain aspects of their behavior if their goals are to be attained, and the consultant must have the ability to facilitate that change. Consultants offer assistance by intervening—that is, by taking some action to solve the problem. These interventions are in the form of learned techniques employed by consultants to address the problem and formulate client problem-solving and decision-making activities.

In Part II the consulting process with its interrelated structure, strategies, and theoretical framework was described. But process knowledge alone does not guarantee successful functioning as a nurse consultant. The consulting process must be effectively applied by the consultant to individual, group, or community clients in a variety of situations and settings. It is now time to consider the equally important topic of how to implement the consulting process. Part III presents guidelines, suggestions, and case studies giving specific intervention strategies for a cross-section of individual, group, and community consultation projects.

The three chapters in Part III focus on different types of clients. Chapter 8 discusses the consulting process as applied to a one-to-one consulting relationship. Individual consulting requires a number of skills and consulting approaches that differ to a degree from group or community consulting. Chapter 8 places emphasis on the common characteristics of individual consulting relationships and on the everyday one-to-one consulting situations that the nurse consultant faces in both internal and external work settings.

Working with groups is the focus of Chapter 9. The group client system is best understood as an indivisible, social, decision-making entity whose actions have a common purpose. Groups involved in consulting endeavors are generally homogeneous in nature—that is, they have a common purpose and orientation. Effective group consultation requires knowledge, skill, and training in group dynamics and group procedures.

Community consultation differs from group consultation in that extreme diversity exists in a community group even though there may be a common goal.

Chapter 10 deals with this diversity of interests, and presents guidelines that assist the nurse consultant to implement effective consulting services in a single, multifaceted situation.

Chapters 8 and 9 contain multiple examples of individual and small group internal and external consultative settings. Chapter 10 concentrates on one in-depth example of a community health consultation, from entry to termination, citing specific task-oriented activities and strategic interventions as they occur.

The chapters in Part III are identically structured. Each moves through the stages of the consulting process from entry to termination, with consultant intervention strategies and application of the theoretical framework interwoven throughout. They are designed to provide the nurse consultant with working models of individual, group, or community consultation.

CHAPTER 8

The Nurse as Consultant to an Individual

One must learn by doing the thing, for though you think you know it—you have no certainty, until you try.

Sophocles

Working with individuals in a consulting situation is perhaps the most demanding type of consultation for both the consultant and the client. The problem area in individual consultation is not as much one of complexity as it is one of high impact or intensity. The intensity of the total relationship revolves around two people, consultant and client, and the problems that they face tend to have more emotional impact than with most group situations. This can be seen in the following typical one-to-one consultation circumstances:

1. Breakdown in the line of communication due to administrator, supervisor, or staff nurse malfunction or incompetence.
2. Immediate choices to be faced that affect future life styles.
3. Dissatisfaction with the present employment situation.
4. A block in the progress of a project due to insufficient knowledge to accomplish the task.
5. Trouble in the work area with an administrator or circumstance.

These are all prime examples of the kinds of situations found when consulting with an individual. Such situations pressure both parties in the relationship to force changes in what may be a relatively short period of time.

All too frequently, clients are forced into an individual consulting relationship because of a crisis situation, often not by their own choice. For example, the internal consultant may be directed by the hospital administrator to help an in-service director plan a new program that she has been reluctant to initiate. In this case neither the consultant nor the client may have requested or desired the involvement, and either one or both may enter the relationship with a reluctance to participate.

Many times, external consultants will also enter consulting situations that are precipitated by a crisis involving an individual in an organizational setting. This can be like being caught between the proverbial "rock and a hard place"—for a period of time nothing seems to work. For the consultant the real crisis is to survive long enough to develop a collaborative relationship with the resentful client. This process takes time and patience, but a collaborative relationship must precede all other efforts. Dinkmeyer and Carlson (1973) point out that this type of a consulting relationship will take more time and more consultant skill to become a productive relationship than almost any other type of consulting endeavor.

Early in any one-to-one consulting relationship, a decision regarding the point of emphasis (behavior or task) must be made. Lewis and Lewis (1977) refer to this decision as the "choice point." They point out that as soon as the specific goal has been clarified and the problems brought to light, the consultant must make a decision regarding the type of change desired for the best possible solution—that is, change in the individual (humanistic) or change in the environment (task). Figure 19 illustrates this first choice point. "Change in environment" in this diagram refers to task orientation and concentration on achieving the stated goal. "Change in individual" is concerned with assisting the individual to break the behavioral and situational cycles that created his or her problems. This is seen as being a necessary and crucial step in many individual consultant–client situations before problem solving can take place and any task achievement can be considered.

This point of emphasis was also demonstrated in a schematic drawing (Fig. 20) by Cory (1963). The illustration clearly shows the inordinate

Figure 19. The first choice point when consulting with an individual. (*After Lewis, J., & Lewis, M. Community counseling: A human service approach. New York: Wiley, 1977.)*

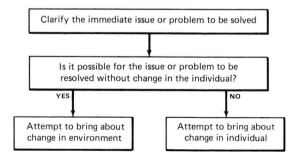

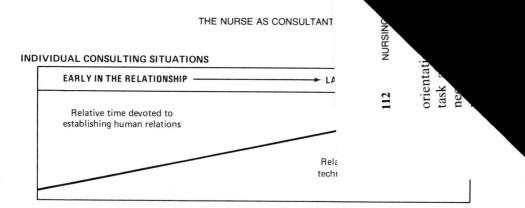

INDIVIDUAL CONSULTING SITUATIONS

EARLY IN THE RELATIONSHIP ⟶ LA

Relative time devoted to
establishing human relations

Rela
techr

MULTIPLE CLIENT CONSULTING SITUATIONS

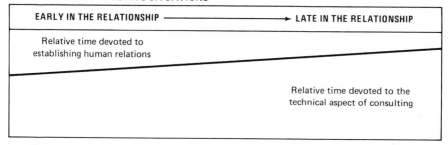

EARLY IN THE RELATIONSHIP ⟶ LATE IN THE RELATIONSHIP

Relative time devoted to
establishing human relations

Relative time devoted to the
technical aspect of consulting

Figure 20. Comparison of the amount of consultant time spent in promoting human relations in individual versus multiple client situations. *(From Cory, S. Helping other people change. Columbus: Ohio State University Press, 1963.)*

amount of consultant time devoted to the area of human relations early in a relationship in a one-to-one client situation as compared to the time spent in multiple client situations.

THE ONE-TO-ONE CONSULTING PROCESS

There are basically three types of individual consulting situations:

1. One-to-one consulting relationship that involves two people (consultant and client) in direct contact with one another.
2. Third-party relationship of consultant–consultee–client in which the consultant collaborates with the consultee, who then in turn collaborates with the client.
3. Consultant working alone in behalf of a client.

The one-to-one consulting process is essentially a learning experience for both consultant and client as they move along a continuum that involves all the consulting components of negotiating, contracting, entry, problem identification, goal setting, problem solving, decision making, action evaluation, and project termination. The major difference in process between individual consultation and group or community consultation is rooted in the on of this type of consulting relationship. In group consultation the always lies in the accomplishment of a common goal. The personal ds of the individual member are of less concern in group consulting, unless a particular member becomes a restraining force to be dealt with before progress toward goal achievement can be resumed. Thus group process is task oriented or environmentally oriented and not so much humanistically concerned with the client's own behaviors. As an example, when a faculty group writes a new school curriculum, the goal or task to be attained obviously bypasses all considerations of group behaviors.

Working with an individual client in a so-called third-party relationship is another common individual consulting situation. This three-way consulting relationship of consultant–consultee–client as used by Caplan (1970), Rogers (1951), and others, is explained in Chapter 3 as the consultee being a professional worker who, after consulting with the consultant, in turn consults with and works directly with the client. A good example of a consultant–consultee–client relationship would be the interaction of a clinical specialist nurse consultant and a staff nurse (the consultee), with the goal being the exploration of problems involved in the nursing care of a particular patient (the client).

The third type of individual consultation is when the consultant works alone on behalf of a client. For example, the nurse consultant may be involved in doing research for a client without ever seeing the client. This is not an unusual situation. Many research surveys are conducted with telephone or mailed reports being the major contact points. In other settings, the consultant may work in the client's environment without a lot of direct involvement.

Another example of a solitary consulting situation—and one that many more consultants will be specializing in—is the area of computerization. Programming educational instruction programs for students or in-service education use, and designing nursing education systems such as patient classification systems, automated care plans, monitoring systems, or quality assurance programs, are examples of common computer endeavors for the nurse consultant (Ball & Hannah, 1984).

STAGE ONE: ENTRY—THE CRITICAL STAGE

The actual time spent in the initial or entry stage (stage one) contact between consultant and client in a one-to-one setting is relatively brief but, as just pointed out, what transpires is surprisingly complex. It is a crucial time because, as compared with group consultation, it is a highly personalized interaction and results in a lasting first impression which is well retained and difficult to erase.

Perhaps the most common emotions felt by the individual client who seeks consultation are uncertainty and anxiety. These emotions are even more exaggerated when the client has no previous experience in a consulting relationship. Thus, consultation is more a personal process in a one-to-one relationship than in either group or community consultation, and the consultant must consider all of the receiving intervention strategies—acceptance, awareness, empathy, encouragement, and genuineness—concerned with promoting effective interpersonal processes. Getting to know the client as a person is often the key to successful or unsuccessful one-to-one consultation. This may require the consultant to be available on an informal level as well as a formal one. For example, taking the time for coffee and lunch breaks has more importance in individual consultations. Obviously, a restaurant is not the place to conduct the business of task accomplishment, but it may be the place where one can break down the early artificial barriers that are sometimes established between consultant and client. The client must believe that the consultant shares his or her concerns and that the consultant is interested in the client as a person, not as an object to be manipulated. Too often the consultant is initially perceived as a personal threat, and the consulting process cannot proceed until this relational difficulty is overcome. The consultant must be sensitive to the client's mind-set and must successfully enter into the client's perceptual field.

The problem with a lack of understanding at this point is that once the consultation reaches the problem-solving and decision-making stages the client may not have the commitment left to cope with all of the problems that emerge. Such an impasse may be strong enough to stop the change process and result in negative consultant–client reactions, with failure to achieve the desired goal.

The quality of the initial interview is thus vital for success. Discussions between the consultant and client must include analysis of what a collaborative consulting relationship involves and what is expected of one another throughout the process. If the consultant has been successful in establishing a quality of human relations that makes effective communications possible, then the task of affecting the change process is greatly facilitated.

Matching consultant skills with the client, wherever possible, is another important aspect of individual consultation that should be realized at the entry stage. Relationships cannot be built on extreme differences. If, for example, the consultant working with a nursing administrator has been in a managerial nursing position, the consultant will know the challenge and will have experienced many of the frustrations of the client. It will be easier to recognize that the administrator's beliefs of "I must be in control" or "I know what is best for the nursing staff" may be major deterrents to the change process. Conversely, the consultant who has only functioned previously in the area of curriculum consultation would find it difficult to understand and work with the many unfamiliar aspects of an administrative situation, and would probably fail to be effective in such a setting.

The Individual Contract

A simple and informal verbal contractual agreement (sometimes referred to as a social contract) is more likely to be the situation in individual consulting than in group or community consultation. A verbal contract is simply an explicit agreement of what the consultant and client expect from each other and how they are going to work together. According to Johnson & Vestermark (1970), a verbal contract is considered legal if it meets four criteria: (1) it was given mutual consent, (2) it received valid consideration, (3) it was freely entered into (no coercion), and (4) it consists of a working agreement about the work to be done and who is to do it.

Problems with contracting are rare when an internal consultant is involved, since he or she is already part of the client's system and readily available. Contracts with external consultants are more often in writing. The written contract does not have to be extensive in form or content. A simple letter or short-form statement of agreement describing the arrangements and signed by both parties is sufficient. Chapter 12 discusses contracting in depth and gives samples of both short-form and long-form contracts.

STAGE TWO: GOAL SETTING

A major role of the consultant during stage two, Goal Setting, is to assist the client to recognize and understand all aspects of the problem, real and implied. This is sometimes difficult when the client does not have support from another individual, family, or group. Although the client might like to "turn the case over" to the consultant, a major role of the consultant is to promote the client's recognition of his or her part in the interaction and to foster the client's awareness of the elements he or she will eventually need to change.

During the initial relationship and interview, the consultant attempts to learn enough about the client and the problem so that the consultant can be more helpful as they enter the second stage. Some questions that need to be answered early include the following:

1. What does the client see as his or her problem?
2. What does the client think needs to be done about it?
3. What has the client already tried to do about it?
4. What does the client expect the consultant to do about it?

It is most important that the consultant and client specifically pursue all aspects of problem identification before attempting to discuss specific interactions related to the problem area.

Encountering Client Resistance

If client resistance is going to occur, it generally happens earlier in a one-to-one consulting relationship than in a group or community setting. This is especially true if an effective client–consultant relationship has not been clearly established during the entry stage. For example, the client might accept the fact that there is a problem, and may even have signed a contract specifying consultant and client roles and responsibilities, without having internalized or fully accepted problem ownership.

In any case, client resistance can be avoided or lessened if the consultant plans for and uses effective intervention strategies, mainly facilitating and energizing at this point. Some additional ways to lessen client resistance, adapted from work by Block (1981) in his book *Flawless Consulting,* are as follows:

1. The consultant should be open and friendly as in any entry session with a client.
2. The consultant should not try to overcome the client resistance with more explanations and pleas for cooperation.
3. The consultant should help the client to express reservations about the consultant and his or her ability to help.
4. The consultant should openly admit that the client has a problem and that he or she wants to help.
5. The consultant should be truthful and give his or her opinions as to the problem and its causes.

Block further points out that if the consultant does all this and still finds resistance and rejection, then the consultant should back off and reassess if the real need has been identified and whether the right services are being or can be offered. There are times when the consultant may have no option except to refuse a contract if there appears to be no possibility of success in the endeavor.

The consultant generally has an easier time handling group resistance than individual resistance. There always seems to be someone in the group ready to help. However, consultants should not progress into the problem-solving or decision-making stages if resistance is not resolved. Some consultants insist on trying to accomplish a task without resolution of disputed points, and sooner or later the entire consulting relationship breaks down. The following is an example of this type of breakdown in a one-to-one consulting relationship.

A consultant is hired by a hospital administrator to work with the director of nursing in a redesign of the nursing administrative structure of the hospital. It is here that the consultant makes an initial mistake by surmising that the established goal is one that the director views positively; in reality the project was "forced" on the director by the hospital administrator and the board of trustees.

Without taking the time to establish a collaborative working relationship, the consultant assumes the "expert" role and pushes ahead with his or her ideas of the changes needed for the redesign of the overall nursing structure, never analyzing the fact that the director of nursing is giving only "lip service" approval to the project. This insensitivity to the real situation results in a gradual build-up of conflict between the consultant and the director of nursing, who now feels the loss of authority, power, and control and begins to work to undermine the project. It doesn't take long for the other nursing personnel to sense the underlying currents of conflict, and they also begin an "underground" of rumors and resistance that leads to dropping the project altogether and dismissing the consultant as ineffective.

The above example is not an uncommon occurrence. The major reason for failure in this case study was an insensitivity on the part of the consultant, combined with a strong need to push the limits of expertise to achieve technical and procedural improvements. This outcome is understandable, but it is important to remember that positive improvement and change is a function of the complex motivation of the client (Cory, 1963). The consultant in this case did not realize that it is the nursing director and not the hospital administrator who provides the consultant with shared power, leadership, and personal support; who schedules the consultant's time; and who provides the physical facilities, supplies, clerical assistance, and so on. In this case, there was a complete breakdown in the major concept of consultation—that is, the true collaboration necessary to ensure that both consultant and client are working together toward the same goal. When such disparity exists consultation cannot be effective.

In addition, when resistance and ambivalence against changing exist, the client will continually attempt to elicit responses from the consultant that are intended to frustrate and distract the consultant and immobilize function. At these times, the consultant needs to examine the client's behavior very carefully for possible cues concerning the characteristic ways that the client copes with threat from significant persons. If these behaviors are understood by the consultant, they will provide clues to how the consultant can counter with intervention strategies that will eventually help the client to acquire a more adaptive response. The task of the consultant here is not task accomplishment but rather to help the client to understand the situation and reach the point of accepting the need for a change of direction. In such a situation, energizing in the form of confrontation as an intervention strategy can be a vital methodology, but it must be implemented with care.

Confrontation, when used appropriately, creates awareness and insight. If inappropriately used it can backfire and result in failure. Remember that many consulting situations requiring consultant use of confrontation are very intense and have a high percentage of consultant failure. Failure by the consultant should not be taken personally. Bell and Nadler (1985) state that not many task-oriented consultants are prepared to deal with destructive resistance. There are times when exiting the consulting situation as gracefully as possible is the only answer available. If premature termination does occur, the client should be referred to other sources, such as another consultant with a strong preparation in therapeutic counseling methods.

Setting Goals

Only after the client problem is defined, driving and resisting forces identified, client resistance overcome, and a collaborative relationship established, can the final step of stage two—setting the goal and subgoals—be accomplished. Target outcomes must be explicitly and objectively defined (see Chapter 5 under Goal Setting). The consultant tries to ascertain what the client wants to change, in what order, and how the client wants to go about it. These questions are all related, ultimately, to the successful identification of the problem solution.

STAGE THREE: PROBLEM SOLVING

Intervention begins with problem solving since, up to this point in the consulting process, the consultant and client efforts have been directed toward establishing a collaborative relationship, defining the problem, and setting goals. What may be lacking now is the client decision to do something about the problem. Acknowledging that there is a problem does not necessitate having a clear understanding of the whole problem or all of its possible effects; deciding to attempt a solution does not imply that there must be a clear idea of what the solution might be or even of how to best approach finding the solution.

The scope, intensity, and urgency of the problem should be considered in establishing a method of attack for the problem. Brainstorming is frequently used for this step. In brainstorming the consultant and client both suggest possible solutions until all ideas have been noted. Even seemingly ridiculous alternatives should be shared and listed; they may be the spark needed to produce a really creative solution. Following a "weeding out" process, the possible realistic alternative solutions should be selected and then analyzed for probability of success, value, and risk using the decision model for analyzing alternative actions (see Chapter 7, Fig. 16).

Some problems require multiple solutions. The process of analyzing alternative solutions does not always result in the choice of a single alternative. But caution should be taken not to choose more solutions than the individual client can handle. The most difficult part of problem solving is to keep the problem and the potential solution in view at all times.

The principle task of the consultant in stage three is to demonstrate to the client the logic of the problem-solving approach, and to teach the client to be his or her own problem-solving analyst. As the client learns the logic by analyzing the alternative solutions to the problem he or she has identified, the client may become increasingly more and more skilled in devising steps to take to reach the desired goal.

STAGE FOUR: DECISION MAKING

Client decision making and taking action toward the final goal achievement, like the problem-solving stage, is no different in individual than in group or community consultation. If the initial entry into the consulting relationship was a good one and all client resistance was overcome by the end of stage two, then the subsequent consulting process should proceed without further impediment. This is not always true of group and especially community consultation, where multiple interrelationships can create many different problems since there are many different individuals involved, creating a constant wave of forward and backward movement in the direction of the consulting process. The one-to-one consulting relationship is much more stable after successful goal-setting and problem-solving stages. Once the decision is made as to the "how" to carry out the various parts of the plan for action, the next step is therefore simply stated: Get on with it.

STAGE FIVE: TERMINATION

Termination with an individual client at times presents some problems to both consultant and client, primarily because of the close interpersonal relationship and dependency bond formed by this closeness. The individual client is frequently more reluctant to initiate independent action and again assume self-direction for the future. The consultant may have to determine the extent to which the client can assume command of his or her own life and whether or not the client will be able to handle similar or other problem situations without consultant help in the future.

The purpose of reviewing the consulting stages and their interplay in a one-to-one consulting relationship is to analyze how they may differ from group or community consultation and to set a stage for the presentation of case studies and specific examples of one-to-one situations. For the purpose of clarity, the four major settings for nursing consultation as presented in Chapter 2—health services consulting, educational consulting, administrative consulting, and research consulting—are used as the framework for the case presentations.

HEALTH SERVICE SETTINGS

Individual health services consultation, also referred to as clinical consultation, like all other forms of consulting is "shared decision making." The consultant responds in the form of intervention strategies to another person's words and needs in such a way that the person can identify a goal and a path leading to that goal. In a clinical nursing situation the client may be any individual (patient, family member, staff member, administrator, or other allied health professional) seeking change in any nursing situation. Some examples of health service settings demonstrating the use of specific consultant intervention strategies follow:

1. A patient faced with a decision to be made regarding a choice of treament or therapy (informing strategy).
2. A family member worried about the cost of hospitalization and needing direction for making financial arrangements (informing and facilitating strategies).
3. A staff nurse troubled about what he or she perceives as an unreasonable work load and requesting help from the internal consultant (receiving, energizing, and reflecting strategies).
4. A home health care agency administrator requesting that the consultant do a utilization review that would reveal gaps in services and then work with staff on recommendations for improved patient care and staff efficiency (receiving, informing, facilitating, energizing, and reflecting strategies).

It should be noted by reading these examples that the extent of the consultant's involvement and the strategies he or she will use depend on the purpose and extent of the service requested. There are times, however, when even the so-called simplest request for information can evolve into a multifaceted consulting situation.

The health services consultant is essential to nursing practice especially in the area of staff support. It seems logical that the internal clinical nurse specialist would be the choice to fill this role in hospitals or other large health care agencies. The consultant role is viewed by Anders (1978), Kohnke (1978), Marcus (1976), and others as a principal role and function of the clinical nurse specialist.

The internal clinical nurse consultant functions daily in many one-to-one consulting situations that generally have two practice components. The first component is directly related to patient care. The preoperative teaching designed to familiarize the patient with the surgical procedure and the coordinating of postoperative care is such an example. The second practice component involves consultation with other members of the health team in a consultant–consultee–client relationship. Here is an example.

Mrs. W., following a radical mastectomy, has a nursing diagnosis of ineffective coping due to fear and lack of acceptance of her impaired body image. She is totally withdrawn and does not respond to nursing interventions developed by the primary nurse. The nurse feels that she needs help with the problem and at this point initiates a request for a nurse consultant.

The request is directed to the oncology clinical nurse specialist who, after the initial consultation with the nurse, in turn decides that the psychiatric clinical nurse specialist is better qualified to handle the immediate problem. A summary of Mrs. W.'s problems is forwarded to the consultant. It is further decided that the nurse requesting the consultation (the primary nurse) will meet with the consultant as consultee acting in behalf of the client (the patient).

The overall goal of the client was to be able to more effectively cope with her medical problem and self-image. The immediate goal of the primary nurse was to find a method to assist Mrs. W. in resolving her problem. The consultant's goal was to assist the nurse in exploring ways to assist the client to effectively resolve the problem.

The initial consultant–nurse discussion was centered on problem solving related to specifying who was the right person to intervene effectively in the client's problem at this point in time. Figure 21 summarizes the situation. An analysis of this decision table did not produce the ideal response of high probability of success, high value, and low cost. Both the nurse and psychiatrist demonstrated high probability of success and high value; but the cost factor was high with the psychiatrist and classified as medium with the nurse, making the nurse the best overall choice.

Once the problem was clearly identified, alternate solutions were evaluated collaboratively and prioritized.

1. Assist Mrs. W. to identify the sources of her stress, anxiety, depression, and withdrawal by:
   - Sitting quietly at her bedside, holding her hand if she will allow it, for a minimum of half an hour in the morning and half an hour in the afternoon.
   - Speaking softly to her and using only short, open-ended questions to encourage her to express her feelings, such as, "Will you tell me what you are feeling right now?"
   - Having her husband follow through with similar verbal and nonverbal communication during his evening visitation.
2. Make arrangements to have someone available at all times to listen to and encourage Mrs. W. to express her feelings if she begins to respond.

Problem: Who should intervene initially with the problem of Mrs. W.'s ineffective coping?			
	Probability of Success	Value	Cost
Nurse	High	High	Medium
Doctor	Medium	High	High
Psychologist	High	High	High
Husband	Low	Low	Low
Mother	Low	Low	Low

Figure 21. Analysis of the problem using the decision-making model.

3. When Mrs. W. is able to discuss her problems freely, assist her to identify and choose alternatives for solving her problem (use the same decision-making table as shown in Figure 16 in Chapter 7 to clarify alternatives).
4. Assist Mrs. W. to identify support systems within the environment, such as family, friends, and the Reach for Recovery program, that can aid her in coping with her problems.
5. Make referrals to appropriate agencies if necessary.
6. Evaluate Mrs. W.'s progress at appropriate intervals even after hospital discharge.

This use of an internal consultant is a valuable adjunct to nursing care in clinical nursing situations that present problems beyond the particular staff nurse's knowledge or experience. The professional, competent nurse recognizes his or her limitations, seeks appropriate consultation, and learns from the findings and recommendations of the consultant.

The external consultant's involvment with a one-to-one direct services consultation is very limited, mostly because of high cost and limited consultant availability for this purpose. If utilized at all by a health agency, the purpose is directed towards upgrading the efficiency of the agency by providing consulting services directly to the administrator, as covered later in this chapter in the "Administrative Settings" section.

EDUCATIONAL SETTINGS

All aspects of consultation involve education of the client to some degree. Thus it is difficult to separate health services consulting and administrative consulting from an educational categorization. When working with an individual client, the consultant can play a vital role in bringing to bear the learning process critically and creatively depending on the situation and the need. In this manner the consultant may be a designer of learning experiences or a direct teacher.

Perhaps one of the best examples of an educational consultant interaction with an individual client is a nurse educator assisting a failing nursing student to change a career goal. The initial intervention strategy here is one of receiving (reviewing facts and listening).

Consultant: I notice that your grades in chemistry, physics, and math are much higher than those in anatomy, physiology, microbiology, and nursing. Do you like those areas particularly?

Student: Yes, I do. I really enjoyed those courses and love to work with figures, but my mother, sister, and aunt are all nurses and they want me to be one, too.

At this point the consultant takes the initiative and enters into an exploration of the problem.

Consultant: What would you choose to be if you had a choice?

Student: I don't know. Probably a bank clerk or an accountant if I can get through college.

Consultant: Your college grades in this area certainly reflect your ability to do so. Have you ever talked to your parents about being an accountant?

Student: Once or twice, but they felt that I would be a long time getting a job in that field, while I can work as a nursing assistant to help out now.

Consultant intervention moves on to informing and facilitating.

Consultant: Did you ever explore part-time jobs in clerking or apprentice accounting at the university placement office?

Student: No I haven't (*smile*). Do you really think there might be a possibility?

Consultant: I don't know, but it is worth looking into. I will give you a referral to Mr. J., with the placement office, and I will call him and let him know you are coming. In the meantime, discuss your concerns with your family, and if they have any questions I will be glad to speak with them on the telephone or arrange an appointment with you and your family.

The nature of the consultant's interventions is clear in this particular example. The initial receptive mode of listening allows the student to express underlying desires. Subsequently, the consultant provides the student with information that facilitates a new action and provides the needed stimulus for planned change. Consultant intervention strategies move in a fairly logical order from receiving to informing and facilitating. Energizing strategies are not used, since the need for confrontation is implied but not needed to force a decision. Reflecting strategies would come later when the consultant again contacts the student and the placement manager to evaluate the success or failure of the intervention.

ADMINISTRATIVE SETTINGS

Administrative consulting also takes two forms: the internal consultant who provides help to individual staff outside the realm of direct services, and the external consultant who is hired to provide consultation directly to a nursing administrator or high-level nursing manager.

In the first instance, the nursing service staff consultant is in a unique position to help individual nurses deal with and resolve their work-related problems. As an internal consultant he or she is available to the staff nurses on an ongoing basis, and is particularly useful to them through not being part of the hospital line authority and having no direct management responsibility. For example, nurses—including those in management positions—seek consultant help for their problems of stress, employer–employee conflicts, ethical dilemmas, personal concerns, medical questions, and so forth. The consultant provides them with the opportunity to express their feelings and helps them use the system in order to solve their problem. In this type of situation it is important that the consultant guarantee confidentiality for nurses with sensitive problems. The client needs to be assured that nothing confidential or personal will ever be revealed.

In the second instance, the external nurse consultant is hired by a higher administrator, such as a board of directors, president or vice president of the hospital, or hospital administrator, to assist in solving an existing administrative problem. The problem may be that there is temporarily a sudden influx of work that needs an extra pair of "expert" hands. The implementation of special projects also frequently calls for consultant assistance. These types of consulting situations are relatively uncomplicated. Helping administrators to solve their own internal or interpersonal problems can be another matter entirely.

Previously in this chapter, the situation of the consultant hired by a hospital administrator to work with a nursing director having major staff problems was cited as an example of client resistance and rejection. In this example, the nurse consultant failed to achieve a successful relationship with the client. But now, assuming that the consultant was able to establish a collaborative relationship, we need to take a look at the subsequent steps involved in problem solving and goal attainment.

Once the client begins to perceive the consultant as a positive rather than a negative force, the client is able to generate objective data that can be analyzed. One of the best methods of obtaining objective data from an individual client without the face-to-face interview and subsequent personalized interpretation is keeping written or taped anecdotal records of consultee behavior by both consultant and client. Prescott (1957) developed the following characteristics for a good anecdote:

1. It gives the date, time and situation in which the action occurred.
2. It describes specific actions of the client, the reactions of other people involved, and the client's response to these reactions.
3. It quotes what is said by the client and others during the action.
4. It supplies "modes cues"—posture, gestures, voice qualities and facial expressions that give clues to how the client felt and reacted. It does not provide interpretations of client feelings, but only the cues by which the reader may judge what they were.
5. The description is extensive enough to cover the episode.

When the nursing director is able, in collaboration with the consultant, to examine the connections between the described personal behavior and the nursing staff's reaction, problem solving starts and constructive alternative actions will begin to fall into place, resulting in progress toward the successful attainment of the overall goal of improvement in communications and interpersonal relationships at all levels.

RESEARCH SETTINGS

The design, direction, and involvement in research is part of the job expectation of the internal consultant. Such research activities are rarely carried out on a one-to-one basis. On the other hand, the external consultant is frequently involved in solitary research activities conducted for a client with no inside or outside assistance. Survey research is a good example of this.

Survey research can be either descriptive or experimental in nature. Descriptive surveys are chiefly concerned with producing as accurate a picture as possible of the real-world situation. Descriptive survey techniques might involve the technique of random sampling, decision trees, linear programming, and risk analysis, to name just a few—all directed toward describing the program itself from the perspective of the provider or service recipient. A survey conducted to describe a Positive Maturity Program's effectiveness would be an example.

Another type of research, required mainly by directors of small health-care agencies, is the small experimental design study, which can provide an unequivocal answer to the ultimate research question: Did the program make any difference or is there a better way to do things? The following example illustrates an experimental study conducted to obtain a better understanding of the effectiveness of a particular method of patient contact.

The director of a community sickle cell project observed over time that the clinic protocol of sending a standard letter informing persons with positive sickle cell tests required numerous followups, mailings, and in many cases two or three telephone calls in order to get a response. A nurse consultant—an expert in community agency functioning—was engaged to assess and provide recommendations to make the process more efficient.

The nurse consultant felt that the project lent itself to an experimental design as to whether (1) the original letter, (2) an improved letter, or (3) home visiting by a nurse (contracted with a home health agency) would be more effective in attracting people to the clinic for further intervention. The study was carried out over a three-month period of time. Whether a person with a positive test result received an original or revised letter, or was visited by a home health nurse, was based on a sequence of random numbers from a standard random number table with a third of the population at risk assigned to each of the three methodologies.

Data were collected by the agency secretary and forwarded by mail to the nurse consultant so that consultant time and agency monies spent on the project were kept to a minimum. After the three-month period, the data were analyzed. It was not suprising that the home visit brought in the highest number of contacts (75 percent). What was surprising was that the improved letter had almost as high a percentage return (66 percent) with the added advantage of a much lower cost to the agency. The original letter had only a 38 percent return. The end result was that the agency did elect to use the revised letter and follow-up with a home visit only on the nonrespondents. (Ideas for case study data were partially drawn from material in Veney and Kaluzny, 1984.)

Other examples of involvement with research as a role function of the consultant include the planning and design of a research project for others to carry out, the actual collecting of the research data, analysis of research data, and report writing of research findings.

SUMMARY

As a unit of change, the individual client is just as important as the group or community client. Walker (1980) points out that probably the oldest technique used by management to improve overall company or agency accomplishment is to improve individual performance. Nurse consultants are frequently utilized to assist clients and consultees (individual nursing administrators, unit managers, and staff nurses) to solve problems and learn techniques that can be made to work more effectively than those already being used.

One of the basic problems encountered by the nurse consultant in appraising individual performance in a large hospital organization is when there is a dual purpose such as personnel performance evaluation as well as program development involved in the appraisal. On one hand, the client (the hospital board of directors or administrator) needs objective evaluation of past individual performance of the director of nurses; the director of nursing needs it on the unit managers; the unit managers need it on the nursing staff; and so on. On the other hand, the same people need tools and techniques to enable all levels of hospital nurses to improve performance, plan future work, develop skills and abilities for career growth, and strengthen the quality of their relationship as employees. Multifaceted involvement can be a complex problem. It occasionally happens in third-party consultation that the consultant is caught between clients and finds it difficult to serve both as judge and consultant. Any consulting contract that involves both evaluation of a client as well as development of the project clearly requires careful consideration and a well-defined purpose, focus, method, and responsibility before contract acceptance.

Nurse consultant services in clinical, educational, administrative, and research settings follow step-by-step progressions along the spectrum of consultant–client relationship. The consultant intervention strategies of receiving, informing, facilitating, energizing, and reflecting, as outlined in this text in a number of examples, are very broad and very general. Nevertheless, they are as vital to all one-to-one relationships as they are to group or community consultation.

SELECTED REFERENCES

Anders, R. Program consultation by a clinical specialist. *Journal of Nursing Administration,* 1978, *11,* 34–38.

Ball, M., & Hannah, K. *Using computers in nursing.* Reston, Va.: Reston Publishing Company, 1984.

Bell, C., & Nadler, L. *Clients and consultants.* Houston: Gulf Publishing Company, 1985.

Block, P. *Flawless consultation: A guide to getting your expertise used.* San Diego: Distributed by University Associates, 1981.

Caplan, G. *The theory and practice of mental health consultation.* New York: Basic Books, 1970.

Cory, S. *Helping other people change.* Columbus: Ohio State University, 1963.

Dinkmeyer, D., & Carlson, J. *Consulting: Facilitating human potential and change processes.* Columbus: Charles Merrill, 1973.

Johnson, D., & Vestermark, M. *Barriers and hazards in consulting.* Boston: Houghton-Mifflin, 1970.

Kohnke, M. *The case for consultation in nursing.* New York: Wiley, 1978.

Lewis, J. & Lewis M: *Community counseling: A human service approach.* New York: Wiley, 1977.

Marcus, J. Nursing consultation: A clinical specialty. *Journal of Psychiatric Nursing,* 1976, *14,* 29–31.

Prescott, D. *The child in the educative process.* New York: McGraw-Hill, 1957.

Rogers, C. *Client centered therapy.* Boston: Houghton-Mifflin, 1951.

Veney, J., & Kaluzny, A. *Evaluation and decision making for health services programs.* Englewood Cliffs, N.J.: Prentice-Hall, 1984.

Walker, J. *Human resource planning.* New York: McGraw-Hill, 1980.

CHAPTER 9

The Nurse as Consultant to a Group

You can measure the efficiency of a group problem-solving session by how fast you reach what seems the best possible solution.

Edward Hodnett, 1959

Much of the critical work of a nurse consultant takes place in group meetings. There are all kinds of groups: families, teams, councils, units, departments, committees, conferences, directors, administrators, faculties, classes, and professional health service agencies, to name a few. Consulting groups can also be classified according to their setting—such as service, educational, administrative, or research oriented. The consulting business functions almost entirely on the basis of group discussion. It is not unlikely that a consultant will give more time to meetings during the course of a consulting contract than to any other form of communication.

In small group consultation, the focus is on the task to be accomplished. This approach is in contrast to that of a therapeutic group, where focus is on each group member and on changing each individual's behavior. Centering on the task or goal does not necessarily eliminate attention to the unique needs, readiness, or motivation of individual group members, especially since the activity of a task-oriented group can be blocked by just one member who holds strong controversial ideas about how to achieve the identified group purpose. For this reason alone an understanding of group theory and function is an area of vital importance to any consultant.

This chapter provides an overview of the theoretical basis of small group theory, identifies characteristics of consulting groups, and discusses the styles and roles of the nurse consultant in implementing the group consulting process. Numerous examples of small group situations are included. These examples provide specific help to the nurse consultant on various aspects of small group interaction as consultation progresses through the stages of the consulting process.

LINKING SMALL GROUP THEORY TO PRACTICE

In every group regardless of its size, shape, or reason for being, reciprocity exists between the members and some degree of mutual aid occurs. People join groups to accomplish something they want or need. To be effective, the consultant must understand the group's purpose and performance.

According to Wilson (1985) the purpose of small group consultation is the encouragement of each individual toward autonomous achievement of concentration on a predetermined goal. In the light of the goal, the consultant and group members work toward some concensus on the desired result. The consultant must take responsibility for understanding how people function in groups and how the group itself performs and develops. Further, the consultant must exercise judgment, intuition, and timing in developing and integrating the consulting process.

Each group has characteristics unique to that particular membership, and each group has a special life and meaning of its own. Yet every group has similar dynamics and follows an identifiable process in its unfolding. There are many variables that distinguish one group from another. The most significant according to Eriksen (1977) are the group's purpose, composition, structure, and function.

Group Purpose

The group's purpose is to accomplish a task set by the group itself or by a higher authority. In order to get the work done and accomplish the task, the group must interact as a unit to explore the problem, identify goals and subgoals, solve the problem, and decide on the course of action. Thus as individual group members interact and develop a sense of interdependence, the group as a whole begins to coalesce and move toward goal achievement. The consultant is the catalyst or facilitator of information processing and the energizer that makes the process work.

Group Composition

The key concept of small group composition is that of "cohesion," which refers basically to the complex forces that bind members of a group to each other and to the group as a whole. These forces identified by Dinkmeyer and Muro (1979), Shaw (1976), and Shepherd (1969) include the satisfaction members gain from being in a group, the degree of closeness and warmth they feel for each other, the pride they feel from being members of a group, the ability they have to meet the task that may confront them as a group, and the willingness to be frank and honest in their expression of ideas and feelings.

Group Structure
The group's structure here refers to the roles and relationships established among members as well as the responsibilities each member is willing to assume to further the group's interests. In using the concept of Lewin's force field theory (discussed in Chapter 7) as a method of analyzing a small group, the consultant will be concerned with those factors that tend to create greater or less cohesion (agreement on goals, tasks to be accomplished, and so on) and those patterns of behavior that result from varying degrees of cohesiveness. The consultant uses his or her own observations as a guide for appropriate intervention. For example, if a member introduces an issue that the group is not ready to deal with effectively due to lack of enough cohesiveness within the group, the consultant may choose to focus the interaction in a safer and less threatening area, or may elect to confront the group with its unwillingness to work on resolving the issue.

Group Function
Small group functions have been viewed by some classic researchers from a developmental sequence viewpoint (Bach, 1954; Bales, 1950; Schutz, 1958; Tuckman, 1965). Tuckman offered a model proposing four general stages as conceptualization of change in relation to group behavior. These stages reflect both social and task realms and are applicable to all group settings. The stages are as follows:

- *Testing and dependence.* This initial group stage is characterized by (1) an attempt by group members to discover and test what interpersonal behaviors are unacceptable to the group based on the reactions of the consultant and on the reactions of the other group members, and (2) by a strong expression of dependency needs by the members toward the consultant, whereby attempts are made to structure the unknown and to find their position in the group. This first stage of task activity development is a time marked by indirect attempts to discover the nature and boundaries of the task—that is, what is to be accomplished and how much work is demanded.
- *Intragroup conflict.* In intragroup conflict the group members react emotionally to the task as a form of resistance to demands of the task on the individual. There exists a defensiveness and resistance where group members clash with one another. This is followed by a phase of "working through anxieties."
- *Development of group cohesion.* An in-group consciousness is now developed and the establishment and maintenance of group boundaries is emphasized. Emphasis is on group cohesion. Now members

accept the group and accept the idiosyncrasies of fellow members. The group becomes an entity by virtue of its acceptance by the members, their desires to maintain and perpetuate it, and the establishment of group-generated norms to insure the group existence.

- *Functional role-relatedness.* The final stage of group development is viewed as the therapeutic stage of understanding, analysis, and insight. It is at this final stage that we observe constructive attempts at successful task completion along with constructive self-change of individual group members.

Thus group process, like the consulting process, works its way from entry to termination. As the group becomes a functional instrument for dealing with the task, the consultant role is that of leader, coordinator, interpreter, informer, and energizer. The relatively short life of a consulting group imposes the requirement that the problem-solving, decision-making, and action-taking stages be reached quickly. The possibility of such rapid development is aided by the impersonal and concrete nature of a task-oriented group. Orientation to the newness of the task is still required, but is minimized by the task rules that preclude much of the emotionality and resistance that are major features of therapy-group development. The more impersonal task and goal-directed group often proceeds without encountering the stage of emotionality as described in Tuckman's stages of intragroup conflict. The exchange of relevant information is also limited by the nature of the task and time considerations in a group. Time involved for a consulting group can be cut to a minimum by a knowledgeable and experienced consultant.

CHARACTERISTICS OF CONSULTING GROUPS

A consulting group is defined here as a small group of ideally five to ten people who interact to accomplish a mutual goal. This definition assumes that the group members interact on a regular basis and have a highly defined structure, such as a formal membership list, specific roles and authority levels (administrator, head nurse, staff nurse; a family structure of father, brother, sister; or the like), and special goals such as increasing their knowledge and skills in a specialty or making a decision on some important group matter. Thus, a consulting group would be classified as a primary group—that is, one in which members are either well known to each other or have common interests and concerns. For example, each member of a particular nursing school faculty is likely to know all of the other group faculty members and to be aware of their specialties and interests. Likewise, a pediatric nurse practitioner joining a previously unknown group of other pediatric nurse practitioners would still have like interests and concerns and would not feel out of place in such a group. Both of these are examples of primary consulting groups. Other examples of primary groups include a family, a head nurse group, an elementary school teacher group, a public health nursing group, and a home health agency group.

The classification of a group as a primary task group (as opposed to a therapeutic group or a therapy group) provides a convenient way to identify the group structure and purpose of any group the consultant might work with. Table 9 provides a more meaningful summary of a task-oriented group in terms of purpose, membership, and leadership characteristics.

STYLES AND ROLES OF THE GROUP CONSULTANT

For the consultant, style, role, personality, and method are invariably inter-related. Of these factors, the consultant probably finds that personality will blend style and method in one way or another. For example, the consultant who identifies group antagonism or overall lack of group support will probably find some refuge in the extremes of a passive or an authoritarian manner in the early contact meetings (in such a setting, the consultant is most likely to act out the role of expert or authority figure). On the other hand, the consultant who senses a positive, warm, and cooperative response from the group will achieve an early self-assurance and develop a natural, persuasive style of encouraging group members to autonomous problem solving and subsequent decision making. The consultant needs to take the time early in the relationship to promote feelings of acceptance and warmth wherever possible.

However, it is well to remember that consultants and their groups do not always "fit." This problem of fit is a challenging one for the consultant, but it is also wise to realize that there are times that relinquishing the

TABLE 9. THE PURPOSE, MEMBERSHIP, AND LEADERSHIP CHARACTERISTICS OF THE TASK-ORIENTED GROUP

Purpose	Accomplish Designated Task
Membership characteristics	Members assigned or volunteer for job Members have common interests and concerns Members are aware of their duties within the group context
Consultant role	Facilitates progress toward desired goal Maximizes problem-solving and decision-making capabilities of the group
Requirements for consultant	Knowledge of task Experience in group leadership Acceptable to members

Adapted from McCann-Flynn, P., & Heffron, B. Nursing from concepts to practice. Bowie, Md.: Robert J. Brady Company, 1984, p. 585.

consultant role to another consultant with more experience and capability in handling a particular group problem is the preferable action and should not be viewed as a personal failure. The suitability of a given group for a specific consultant is often unpredictable before initial group sessions. The degree and quality of the consultant–group contact is crucial for building the structure for goal attainment. An ineffective consultant will only tend to become controlling and obtrusive, thus upsetting the balance and inhibiting client autonomy and independence.

Group resistance that emerges from a build-up of unexpressed individual or subgroup distractions can sap the life and vitality of the group. Any resistance readily takes the form of a counter group work force whose time is spent in "putting down" the consultant. In such an antagonistic group, the consultant symbolizes an oppressive authority and is generally ignored or harassed. The following illustration demonstrates how one such resistant group member galvanized others into expressing distrust, defensiveness, and hostility toward the consultant.

> A number of intensive care staff nurses were consulting with a clinical specialist about improving the group's poor communication and interpersonal relationship skills. One nurse, unable to tolerate critical references to the ongoing, here-and-now group process, refused to talk about what the group's problems actually were. Instead she wanted to talk about her work experiences and accomplishments. She persistently accused the consultant and other group members of bringing forth problems that she had no part in (thereby denying the very basis of the reason for the meetings). She further challenged the consultant's authority by defending several participants whom she felt were "unfairly" called on for "personal" feelings about their work.
>
> Other group members, disgruntled with the unfairness in their working arrangements, also displaced their hostility about the system onto the consultant. Adding fuel to the fire was the consultant's air of formality, aloofness, and reticence to discuss the problem with the group. The consultant's attitude gave surface credence to the speculation that the consultant had been secretly imposed upon the group by the administration as an authority figure. After several sessions of this kind, the consultant decided with the group that no further progress was possible. The group was disbanded and the consulting contract voided.

In retrospect the consultant realized that she was not the right person to handle this situation and that this was not the time, place or group for defusing such massive resistance. The consultant wisely withdrew, and strategically admitted to a momentary but not lifelong defeat.

All consultants are confronted with problems—some serious, many not so serious—and somehow most of them are resolved. When disruptions first begin to occur within a group, it is important for the consultant to have a repertoire of responses in order to maintain control and to accomplish the objectives of the meeting. Jones (1980) identified several responses that can be used effectively to prevent attempts by individuals to dominate meetings at the expense of the consultant. These include:

1. Give the disruptor a special task or role in the meeting, such as summarizing the viewpoints of others.
2. When a disruptor has been previously identified, arrange an individual meeting to work out differences, possibly with a third party facilitator.
3. Get the disruptor's cooperation for the next meeting. Ask the person to agree not to argue from a fixed and often familiar position.
4. Structure the meeting to include frequent discussion and presentations by other cooperative members.
5. Take all of the disruptor's items off the agenda.
6. Set the person up to be concerned about what might be the consequences of disruption. For example, "It has come to my attention that a number of people are angry with you, and I am thinking about opening up their discussion at the meeting."
7. Set up other persons who will tend to support you in dealing with the disruptive behavior of the individual. For example, they can be asked to refuse to argue with the person, give feeling reactions to the dominating behavior, or confront the dysfunctional behavior directly.
8. Make the person's behavior a published agendum (p. 162).

All of these methods require that the consultant adopt a cool, unruffled posture. Keeping control of the situation and not becoming angry usually provides the best outcome for maintaining control during the meeting itself. Remember that people who attempt to dominate have energy that can sometimes be channeled productively, and the best outcome would be that the disruptor becomes an effective meeting participant. Style and method are individualized consultant characteristics, and with training and experience can be used effectively in most group consulting situations.

FACILITATING THE ENTRY STAGE

At the onset of a consulting group, regardless of consideration and contractual arrangements made prior to the first session, there will be a certain amount of confusion about the nature of the task, the role of the group members, and the responsibilities of the consultant. This entry stage is a crucial one and the effective consultant must be able to clarify the purposes of the group, clearly establishing the fact that the group is to be involved in a collaborative relationship involving problem identification, goal setting, problem solving, decision making and evaluation (including termination). Obviously when working with groups the consultant's job is simultaneously doubled and divided, because a group is a multi-client situation, and the consultant needs to be especially attentive since there will be many interactions taking place at the same time. The consultant must be able to actively facilitate the group's goals. To do so the consultant must recognize and, when appropriate, respond to the members who initiate, contribute, elaborate, provide information, and offer or seek opinions. Making group members aware of their own strengths and assets in being able to effectively work through the problem-solving and the decision-making process is an early major focus of group consultation.

Perhaps group facilitation by the consultant can best be demonstrated in the example of a consulting group of nursing faculty who have as a common goal the adoption of a new curriculum. But faculties are generally made up of a diverse group of people coming from a variety of clinical backgrounds and educational experiences, and can hold radically different ideas on what the curriculum should be and how it should be implemented. It takes a great deal of consultant skill to maintain the task focus and at the same time assist the individual group members to confront, encounter, and clarify each other's affective and cognitive domains and perceptions, and to help mold and change beliefs, attitudes, and behavior constructively.

The consultant serves as a facilitator of action and change. The steps involved in achieving group cohesion are very much a function of how the consultant develops leadership in the group. In consultation, it stands to reason that the best leader is the one who helps the group achieve their desired goal. To do this the consultant, early on, needs to help the group examine the following ideas:

1. What common goal exists among group members?
2. What can they expect from the consultant as a leader?
3. What help does the group need?
4. What can the group members expect from each other?
5. What limits does the group wish to set on members' behavior?
6. What limits exist that set boundaries on group actions and goals?

During the entry stage, one way for the consultant to demonstrate concern for the group is by providing members with frequent opportunities to express their feelings and problems. Typically groups start by expressing their insecurity over unclear boundaries. For example, a common question would be: "Are we supposed to accept the new curriculum guidelines or can we change them to meet the needs as we might view them?" From the very beginning, the group will need to test out the consultant's reactions to its needs. The earliest needs to appear in the group will be those of dependency–interdependency, agreement–hostility, and the need for acceptance by both the consultant and the group. Part of the consultant's initial job will be to develop in the group sources of security to meet any threats. By pointing out the differences in feeling and points of view among group members, and by showing how different members are expressing similar concerns, the consultant helps the members see their common goal and problems. This approach facilitates identification between members.

Coordinating Group Activities

The initial leadership role of the consultant is a "linking" or coordinating function. The consultant makes an effort to perceive the linkage between the separate comments of the group members, and conveys this relationship to the group, so that the discussion then seems to flow as one current that builds up force as each new contribution is linked to it.

The linking function of the consultant is closely related to the strategy of reflecting (consultant intervention strategies were described in Chapter 6) the meanings of group members' statements. This is because the meaning of a group member's comment often is the link to goal clarification and overall purpose of the consulting relationship. The consultant is not only the reflector and the facilitator who makes clear the meaning and purpose of the group but also provides the force that activates the group to move onward toward specific goal setting, problem solving, decision making, and action. All consultant intervention strategies must be employed in the appropriate segments of group life. For example, Egan (1970) stresses the fact that even when faced with initial group resistance, confrontation too early in the life of the group could harm rapport and hinder group cohesion.

The physical problems of keeping a group together, even in the entry and goal-setting stages, can have a significant bearing on cohesion in the group and thus on the overall potential of the group to clearly define its problem and set realistic goals. Many attendance problems can be avoided by early careful planning and scheduling and by establishing effective devices for communication about group activities. The consultant should check the schedules of all participants to determine the best possible meeting times, making sure that an appropriate room is available, and establishing and sending out agendas before the meeting.

Remember that it is impossible to develop or sustain a high energy level in groups where members are uninterested or uncommitted to the goal. Enthusiasm and the ability of the consultant to involve all members in the group process is a critical factor in assuring that a consultant group will have a high energy level. The capacity of the consultant to stimulate a group through his or her own behavior is an important skill. Role modeling of the consultant by the client cannot occur until the consultant "has modeled her client's world and has aggregated and analyzed the constructions of that world" (Erickson et al., 1983, p. 95).

Developing Ground Rules

Every group sets up ground rules for the nature and intensity of its interactions. These ground rules include the fairly simple tasks of setting time and place of the meetings to the more involved questions of acceptable and unacceptable behavior of individual members within the group. Often the consultant is involved in these activities, but it is highly desirable for members of the group to take the leadership role wherever possible. This clearly establishes, from the start, that members themselves have a primary responsibility for the group. To a degree, involvement in the routine work of the group is an indicator of commitment to the total project.

Behavioral ground rules for group members should be specific as to what is acceptable or unacceptable bahavior. For example, a faculty group implementing a new curriculum may decide not to permit its members to discuss personal feelings or issues about the already accepted curriculum design. When the ground rule is broken, the consultant should point it out, so that the group can avoid unnecessary digressions. Ground rules are often included in the group's written contract, but sometimes also surface later and need to be added. The consultant needs to be alert to this possibility and to bring it to the group's attention for discussion and resolution.

There are several unwritten ground rules that usually apply to all groups. They include the fact that members are generally expected to listen to each other, to respond to each other, to be relevant in their comments, and to give "equal time" to all members. When these interactional rules are not followed, friction or discomfort results within the group, and it is the consultant's responsibility to confront and correct the situation so that the group can proceed with its tasks.

Confidentiality in Groups

It is probably unrealistic to expect that information disclosed in a consultation group—especially in a large group—will always be kept in confidence. For this reason group participants may be reluctant to discuss situations involving material that may be personally embarrassing or damaging if divulged outside the group.

Because of the possibility of sensitive material being presented (individuals being discussed, and the like), the problem should be broached by the consultant near the beginning of the group discussion. The group itself should set norms on confidentiality and must decide what materials will be kept in confidence. From the outset of consultation it must be evident that the goal of consultation is to make effective change, and that this is collaborative in nature and carefully planned. This approach is a major deterrent to a negative impact on the consulting group. When the group itself claims ownership of the data being exchanged, confidentiality generally does not become a problem.

TASK ACCOMPLISHMENT AND THE GOAL-SETTING STAGE

Consulting groups are organized for a purpose—that is, to accomplish a goal that is acceptable to all group members and the consultant. A major problem in some groups is that the goals of the consultant and the goals of the group members do not always seem to be in agreement. Sometimes one or more of the group members will still be motivated by personal needs. Such a situation existed in the example given earlier in this chapter of consultant failure when working with a hostile and antagonistic group of intensive care nurses. In such cases, the consultant must be concerned with the conversion of various goals individual members might hold into a common group goal that will be influential enough to initiate group problem-solving activity.

Group goals are also inducing agents that serve to direct group action. Once a goal has been set, all members are expected to work toward that goal even when it is not one selected by an individual member. In essence, the goal of a group, once selected, is a group motivating factor with varying degrees of intensity and influences for different members. As shown by Tuckman's (1965) model of the stages of group activity development (discussed earlier in this chapter under "Group Function"), the motivational properties of groups make it explicit that members who are clearly aware and acceptant of group goals are more likely to cooperate. The individual who either dimly perceives the group goal or is not in agreement with it will tend to be motivated by personal needs. Thus if the purpose is to elicit change, group members must be aware of the purpose of the group, clearly see the expectations, accept some responsibility to change, help others to change, and work at mutual goal achievement.

The goal-setting, problem-solving, and decision-making stages are periods in which the group experiences a sense of cohesiveness and is highly active in pursuing its goals.

METHODS TO FACILITATE GROUP PROBLEM SOLVING

Clients need more than ideas. If they are to change, the consultant must help members to integrate new ideas, make decisions, and take action. According to Dinkmeyer and Carlson (1973) and Dinkmeyer and Muro (1979), the aim of working with groups is not for the consultant to "play expert" but to transfer his or her "expertise" into the working repertoire of others. The consultant who provides all of the answers inhibits any problem-solving activity on the part of the group members, and even if the answer is accepted it will not be internalized and acted upon.

The group's success at problem solving will be greatly enhanced by the consultant's contributions of information about resources and feasible alternative action strategies as well as information about obstacles the group can anticipate from a chosen course of action. The consultant also has the responsibility of helping the group to weigh the practicality (probability of success, risk, and value) of alternative courses of action. Use of the problem-solving model shown in Figure 16 during this stage will, in most instances, graphically clarify the most effective course of action.

However, there are occasions—especially when working with larger groups (seven to ten or more people)—that an unusual number of alternative actions will present themselves, calling for a presorting and weeding-out process before logical decision making can take place. Other techniques for obtaining data and breaking a complex problem into smaller components are available for use. Two of the more efficient techniques for this purpose include specialized versions of the nominal group process and the Delphi technique.

Nominal Group Process

The nominal group process technique was first proposed by Delberg and Van de Ven in 1971 and later improved upon by Green and Petri in 1973. Nominal group technique is used for problem exploration when the group process itself is not sufficient to generate the data and informed judgments required to proceed into subsequent phases of decision making. This technique is a more structured version of brainstorming. The advantages are that it pares down the number of possible alternative actions to a few major ones quickly and effectively, and eliminates interpersonal criticism by individual group members without interfering with overall group interaction.

The process is a simple but carefully structured series of steps. It includes the following briefly summarized procedure:

1. Each group member is asked to rank-order their solutions to the stated problem in a silent generation of possible actions to solve the problem.
2. The proposed actions are then listed on a blackboard or flipchart and categorized according to an assigned priority number. This process continues, without discussion, until all actions have been listed.
3. The consultant next leads the group in a discussion of the recorded ideas for the purpose of clarification, elaboration, and evaluation. Each item is discussed sequentially and no items are eliminated from the list.
4. Each participant, without interacting with others, is then asked to select the ten most important alternative actions on the total list and rank them in order of priority from one to ten (in special cases this could be limited to five).
5. Finally, a group decision is made based on the outcome of the members' individual votes. If indecision still exists, a discussion and then a final secret vote might be indicated.

The Delphi Technique

The Delphi technique is a process of gathering data and concensus while clarifying opinions from individuals without a meeting. In reality it is a nominal group process implemented by mail. It has the advantage of being anonymous but the disadvantage of being time-consuming. It is most effectively used by the consultant following a previous meeting marked by indecision, squabbles, and overall blockage. Taking the time before the next meeting to give individual members the opportunity to express opinions in an impersonal and anonymous setting can provide the impetus needed to get the group back on an effective level of functioning.

The exact procedure in using the Delphi technique may vary depending on the need and anticipated results. Generally the technique as proposed by de Brigard and Helmer in 1970 serves as a method to elicit brief statements regarding the problem solution. Like the nominal group process, possible alternative actions can be rank-ordered.

Theoretically the Delphi technique is a collection and tabulation technique with two or three mailings involved, but for the consultant's purpose a single input if handled well will provide the consensus on data needed to give impetus to meaningful group discussion at the next meeting. According to Gordon and associates (1976) and Pike (1970), one of the Delphi's greatest strengths is its ability to avoid the pitfalls of open, unstructured group discussion—that is, group pressures, an unwillingness to abandon publicly stated opinions, and the effects that individuals have on groups. Additionally, when used with a consulting group facing major blockage problems, it can provide a "cooling down" and introspective period for group members.

Nominal group process and the Delphi technique are not the only group techniques that could be used effectively to stimulate productive group participation and problem solving. According to Fitzgerald and Murphy (1982), the more recent *quality circles* approach as a tool for eliciting ideas, solutions to problems, and recommendations for goal achievement is an equally reliable tool for problem solving. Each consultant, in the course of a consulting career, will develop expertise in many such techniques. It has been the author's experience that the use of these techniques works well as an adjunct to the use of the models proposed in Chapter 7 for facilitating the consulting process.

COLLECTIVE DECISION MAKING

Small, cohesive groups with a common goal and a positive approach toward problem-solving alternative actions for goal achievement possess the capacity to respond and act in an effective manner. Such collective decision making is an outgrowth of collaboration and helps eliminate the possibility of a win or lose situation. It also creates a greater sense of ownership of the ultimate decision by group members.

When there is active group participation in the decision-making process there is usually much more ownership in the decision and action that follow. The motivation to see that goals or tasks are carried through can be greatly enhanced through group action. Also, implementation is not left up to one or two individuals unless clearly designated by the group. Even if implementation is delegated by the group to various members, a strong team member's support is usually present.

Broadening the decision-making base will require that everyone involved move away from the comfort of the traditional one-way decision-making modality (linear) and experience the risk and responsibilities of mutual decision-making. For example, staff nurses on a team planning an interdisciplinary approach to patient education in their unit must become comfortable with broad participation in the decision-making process and recognize that they may need to adjust to the idea that "outsiders" will be part of the team needed to improve the learning environment.

When there is a block in the consulting process and the decision made cannot be implemented, the use of the *model for viewing and analyzing driving and restraining forces* (see Fig. 14) can be helpful. Use of this model requires the group to identify and list the driving (helping) forces, which provide a positive improvement in the situation, and those restraining (hindering) forces resistant to change. The group selects the forces that seem pivotal to the situation and that they may be able to affect. For each of the restraining forces identified by the group as particularly important, the group then lists possible actions that might reduce or eliminate the effect of the force. In addition, for each of the important driving forces the group lists action steps that would serve to increase its effect. In this way a step-by-step program of action is devised that can facilitate effective implementation. This method helps the group solve immediate conflicting problems anytime a block occurs. Perhaps the most important asset lies in the model's ability to graphically display the lists of the driving and restraining forces for client clarification.

TERMINATING THE SMALL GROUP PROCESS

Like everything else, groups reach a point where they end. In the consulting relationship where the contract has been clearly defined, termination should present no major problem. Closure represents a distinctive part of a group's life and goal achievement.

Keeping a group moving efficiently toward the solution of the problem is a consultant's first duty. Small groups, as a general rule, will move faster than a one-to-one consulting process mainly because there are more people to do the work and, once the group gets moving, the momentum accomplishes the tasks in a shorter period of time. The small group is less dependent on the consultant and usually more willing to assume self-direction once the goals have been reached. As Schwartz and Goldiamond (1975) so aptly put it: "The consultation ends when the contracted terminal repertoire is actually the current relevent repertoire of the group and they assume responsibility for it" (p. 128).

SETTINGS FOR SMALL GROUP CONSULTATION

As in individual consulting, group consultation takes place in a variety of health services, educational, administrative, and research settings. The usual circumstances are that a dean of a school of nursing, faculty, director of nursing, hospital administrator, health-care manager, or staff member from a subgroup of a health-related agency seek out the consultant. But no matter what the setting, it is important to always approach small group consultation as an organized process. The successful ingredient in this type of consultation is high client involvement at all stages of the process. Such involvement is the key factor in increasing the group's commitment to work collaboratively for change.

HEALTH SERVICE SETTINGS

Through direct consultation in health service settings, the consultant helps group clients—professional nurses, allied professionals, patients and families—gain the expertise they need to solve a problem and meet a need. The consultant is also in a position to offer suggestions, impart information, and expedite the client's decision-making process by being prepared and by knowing what is expected in light of service to others. The following discussion highlights some of the more common catagories of service settings and provides some examples of consultants at work.

Family Group Consultant
In a hospital setting, the internal consultant is frequently the contact point between the family and the different interaction systems operating in the patient setting. The family group can be viewed as an advice seeker and the consultant as an advice giver. The family is in effect asking "What would you do? What would you suggest to us?" Families frequently need help to define specific problem areas and to identify all of the possible alternative actions for problem solution. One thing the consultant must do is to make sure that all possible recommendations are made and the consequences outlined. The alternate choices should be ordered accordingly in collaboration with the family (and patient), analyzing the probability of success, the risk, and the value for each particular situation (see the example of the analysis of alternative choices applicable here in Fig. 17).

Staff Group Consultant
The internal or external nurse consultant intervenes frequently in the process of monitoring staff concerns and problems. Sometimes meetings are held periodically with various staff groups to do the following:

1. Share concerns about patients, the nursing process, staff relationships, and the nursing environment.
2. Begin to identify the problems in their areas of concern.
3. Learn why these identified problems exist and how they affect their present situation. Identify driving and restraining forces.
4. Learn new procedures for facilitating improvement (e.g., problem-solving alternative actions and planning changes).
5. Give and receive feedback on the implementation of planned actions.
6. Provide for an ongoing communication network.

The following example illustrates staff group consultation. A head nurse on a medical unit requests consultation because he has not been able to intervene effectively in a situation of apparent unrest and distress among the unit nursing staff. He states that the problem started when staff assignments were changed in the hospital, resulting in the transfer of nurses between units. The need for the transfer was precipitated by a shift in patient count and the initiation of some new cost accounting measures. The staff appeared to accept it and understand it at the time, but now staff concerns and problems seem to have multiplied to the point that normal functioning of the unit is disrupted.

Since the request for consultation was initiated by a nurse in an administrative position, the consultant elects to use a modified Delphi technique to collect data from the staff before the first face-to-face meeting. A survey questionnaire eliciting staff concerns and their perceived reasons for the existence of the problems is given to each staff member by the consultant. This personal contact gives the consultant the opportunity to provide explanations to each of the staff nurses about the purpose of the consultation, to arrange the first meeting, and to ensure staff anonymity. Another advantage of this approach is that it enables the consultant to enter the relationship armed with the knowledge, expertise, and preparation the group needed, thus enabling both consultant and group to move more rapidly to the area of concern.

Clinical Nurse Specialist Consultant

The current activities of the clinical nurse specialist involve all three forms of nursing consultation—that is, the expert consultant who has the knowledge and skills to solve the problem, the resource consultant who provides relevant information to enable the client to make decisions based on the widest range of alternatives, and the process consultant who directs and collaborates in all aspects of collaborative problem solving and decision making (Kohnke, 1978).

As a case in point, the use of a nurse consultant on a hospital dialysis unit after the change from functional to primary care was cited in an article by Dean (1979). The decision to hire a consultant to bring about change and improve nursing care was initiated by the unit nurses themselves. However, the consultant employed—although an outsider or external consultant—was well known by all of the employees and respected for her competence and ability as a dialysis nurse and educator. This preexisting acceptance of the consultant greatly facilitated group communication and accounted for the rapidity with which the group made the decisions and adjustments needed to initiate the primary nursing approach.

The use of a clinical nurse in infection control is another example of effective consultant use. In this setting, a nurse consultant with the necessary training and experience to enable him or her to work as an infection control specialist has an important and special contribution to make toward an improved standard of care and to greater safety of patients in hospitals. The consultant in this role is advisor, researcher, and teacher.

School Nurse Consultant

An increasing number of states are appointing a nurse consultant to work with teachers, children, and parents on health-related problems. The consultant usually has advisory and liaison functions in a specific school district and is involved with planning of health education services and policy. Other responsibilities may include the organization of workshops and the coordination of standards of health performance for the children and school personnel. As a specialized school team member, along with the educational psychologist, resource specialist, speech therapist, and other educational experts, the nurse consultant is very much involved with evaluation or audit of school health services (Slack, 1980). It is readily apparent that when viewing group segments of a school setting in terms of direct service that aspects of the educational, administrative, and research functions are involved. The school nurse consultant's position is a multifaceted one in respect to both role and function.

Traditionally the school nurse consultant role has been limited to one of health advisor and health information or health educational coordinator. It is extremely important that the role be expanded to include health team development, human relation approaches, and public relation techniques to promote healthful practices and community development.

The school health nurse consultant has untold opportunities to influence the health concept, learning, and health environment in school settings. Innovative school health programs such as the School Health Curriculum Project (U.S. Department of Health and Human Services, 1977) are being widely implemented throughout the United States. This program is not only comprehensive concerning the subject matter of health and disease, it is also comprehensive in its approach to integrating classroom learning experiences with other life situations and activities and people contacts. The program is a "natural" to build on innovative school nursing programs such as the Project Health PACT (Participatory and Assertive Consumer Training) developed by the University of Colorado School of Nursing (Igoe,

1980). The school nurse consultant is the ideal person to set up a collaborative team to direct the integration of a total school health program.

EDUCATIONAL SETTINGS

Group educational settings involve nurse consultants in a teacher or educational specialist role in schools of nursing, industry, hospitals (in-service and continuing education), and public health and community agencies. Function as a consultant in educational settings rarely involves direct service. A discussion of each of these categories follows.

Schools of Nursing

Educational consulting in a school of nursing most frequently involves the areas of curriculum development and program evaluation. Curriculum consultation consists of all of the planned educational activities within the school environment. It is primarily concerned with determining overall educational goals, selecting appropriate curriculum design (courses and content), developing designs for achieving these goals (including student clinical experiences), and developing specific instructional designs to meet and assess the goals.

Some questions that the curriculum consultant and faculty need to answer before embarking on curriculum design or revision were first proposed in a clinical study by Tyler (1969) as part of his widely accepted four point curriculum model.

1. What educational purposes should the school seek to attain?
2. What educational experiences are likely to achieve these purposes?
3. How can these educational experiences be effectively organized?
4. How can we determine whether the purposes are being achieved?

Saunders and associates (1981), in an article on the role of the curriculum consultant, also provide nursing consultants with some practical guidelines for analyzing a nursing curriculum. They stress the following points:

1. The faculty's philosophy should provide for identifying program objectives and for establishing a conceptual framework.
2. Program objectives must be stated in measurable terms and must be attainable.
3. Objectives should reflect behaviors in the psychomotor and affective domains as well as the cognitive domain.
4. The objectives should clearly identify the competencies for which the student is being prepared.
5. All major concepts must be identified and clearly stated. Subconcepts and theoretical formulations should be specified for each of the major concepts.

6. The vertical and horizontal threads of the curriculum should be identified by the consultant and faculty to determine if continuity, sequence, and integration of learning exist.
7. The level objectives should specify behaviors that students must demonstrate within a designated period of time. These flow from the program objectives and reflect progress in student abilities and skills.
8. Derived from level objectives, course objectives should be specific and should serve as the basis for identifying course content, learning experiences, and evaluation tools.
9. Evaluation must be an integral part of the curriculum planning so that corrective actions can be taken as inadequacies are identified. The evaluation process should focus on the analysis of objectives and content so that each segment can be delineated for evaluation.

More specific guidelines for curriculum design, formulation, and evaluation can be obtained from the NLN and regional accreditation bodies that routinely publish criteria for the establishment and accreditation of nursing programs.

Industrial Consultant
The focus of consultation is often directed toward modifying the physical, psychological, and educational environment of an industrial setting. In an attempt to meet the public demand for more effective health care for workers and their families, industrial administrators are increasingly using the services of nurse consultants who can provide the administrators, their safety and accident prevention teams, and their industrial nurse (if any) with objective counsel and recommendations for ways in which to improve the delivery of industrial health care.

Another aspect of the use of a nursing consultant in industry is that of working directly with companies manufacturing health-related products. A nurse consultant in industry might function in the role of a resource-person for the sales or marketing team in a particular company. Such a nurse might also provide educational service to customers to help them use the products correctly and efficiently. These consultants are a valuable link between manufacturer and product user (Koch, 1979). Generally this type of industrial consulting is as an internal (salaried) consultant. With our ever-increasing health product technology, it is a continuously expanding field for nurse consultants.

In-Service and Continuing Education
Internal and external consultants will receive requests for seminar presentations, formal classes, or workshop and conference presentations from a multitude of health agency, educational, administrative, and research settings. Much of this has been previously covered in Chapter 2 under educa-

tional consulting, particularly in the discussion of the teaching role of the nurse consultant.

Some nurse consultants develop expertise on a specialized level of nursing practice, such as in formulating nursing diagnoses, or in a field of high demand clinical expertise, to a point where lecture engagements, writing, or consultant assignments are highly rewarding. Teaching opportunities for full-time or part-time expert consultants are burgeoning today as various states mandate continuing education requirements for licensure of nurses and as workshops proliferate. Even adult education courses that include aspects of wellness and health promotion as well as prevention and disease control abound in virtually every community. It only takes some concentrated self-marketing by the consultant to establish a reputation in these areas and find opportunities for free-lance teaching.

Public Health and Small Agency Consulting

The increasing public demand for accountability in human services has left almost no program unaffected. The utilization of the nurse consultant as a "core committee" member to plan, implement, and evaluate health-related programs and educational offerings in public health as well as in other health-related agencies is well documented by Koch (1979), Kohnke (1978), McCann and associates (1984), Smiley (1973), and others.

Also, program consultation in health services frequently involves consultant collaboration in the design and development of instrumentation such as reporting forms and instruction manuals to be used by health services professionals. As distinguished from case consultation, program consultation focuses upon the agency's planning, development, organization, and administration of services rather than upon specific problems in serving a client.

ADMINISTRATIVE SETTINGS

Working with small groups of health administrators is another common work setting for the nurse consultant. The administrators can be part of the same agency or be representatives from a cross-section of agencies with similar goals.

One such instance might be the use of a nurse consultant to work with a group of hospital nurse managers or supervisors with a focus and goal of developing administrative personnel who will understand and utilize group dynamics more effectively. The consultant brings to this setting his or her expertise in the roles of leader and teacher.

Consultation to administrative groups is a sensitive and complex undertaking. Certainly, the nurse consultant must be an expert in the field of concern. Consultants who are effective in any setting are those who are able to think while doing, who can respond to presented problems while conceptualizing about larger or related problems, and who are secure enough in their own selves that they can deal with the potential pitfalls and unexpected consequences that inevitably develop in this type of group. The process and problems involved with consultation in small group administrative settings are touched on at a number of points throughout this book.

RESEARCH SETTINGS

Consultant involvement with small group research is so individualistic that it is almost impossible to catagorize. It can run the gamut from helping groups develop and implement their own research designs to the consultant's being solely responsible for the research project on a contractual basis. The three typical case studies that follow demonstrate this diversity.

For the first example, a home health-care agency has been funded to initiate a one year study of the progress and recovery of patients over age 65 with a diagnosis of fractured hips. The study involves the control of many variables such as the types of passive and active range of motion exercises provided, nutritional supplementation, and the number of nursing visits.

Another example would be an industrial plant with an unusually high number of accidents that engages the services of a nurse consultant to assist the health and safety personnel to set up a health clinic to meet their needs. However, before the consultant can proceed to the goal of establishing a health clinic he or she must know and understand all aspects of the problem situation. This requires research into the number and types of accidents occurring in this setting, the locations in which the accidents occurred, and any extenuating circumstances surrounding the accidents. These research data are required to supply not only the information the industry needs to open an industrial health clinic but might also supply the information and stimulus that management and workers must have to set up an accident prevention program as well as a health clinic.

As a third example, a nurse consultant might be engaged to direct and assist a hospital unit nursing staff with the implementation of research designed to identify and study patients with possible nosocomial (hospital-acquired) infections and to oversee it periodically for a six-month period of time. Here the consultant works with the staff involved to direct the research process, but is never directly involved in the clinical data-gathering process.

Descriptive or analytic surveys concerned with gathering as accurate a picture of a group problem area as possible are frequently made by a consultant without the cooperation or coordination of the group's members under study. Another example of such a survey would be a contractual agreement between a consultant and the hospital administration to study the productivity of nurse practitioners and physician assistants. This type of research project would be carried out with the cooperation of the nurse practitioners and physician assistants involved, in the form of self-administered questionnaires or interviews but without the collaboration that makes a joint research project. In this case the consultant's responsibility is only to the administration and not to the study groups.

SUMMARY

In small group consultation, consultants are facilitators of action and change. They encourage, observe, harmonize, help shape group norms, and are generally responsible for promoting optimum group growth.

Another key function of the consultant is role modeling—that is, engaging in those behaviors that will promote the learning process and encourage independent group action. These behaviors range from acceptance to confrontation and include encouragement, self-disclosure, self-examination, expression of feelings, cooperation, and the maintainance of the here-and-now focus. All of these interventions are employed in the appropriate segments of group life.

The most potent aspect of small group consultation is the high level of commitment and the fact that the group itself—once the goal has been identified and accepted—becomes the major motivating factor for goal attainment. The group declares joint ownership of the problem, collaborates with the consultant to problem-solve, and initiates all goal-seeking activity. The consultant provides only the catalytic action needed to stimulate the group to share ideas, become cohesive, and develop in an effective manner. Thus small group consultation with primary or homogeneous groups is perhaps the easiest and usually the most successful of the possible consulting situations.

SELECTED REFERENCES

Bach, G. *Intensive group psychotherapy.* New York: Ronald Press, 1954.

Bales, R. *Interaction process analysis: A method for the study of small groups.* Cambridge, Mass.: Addison-Wesley, 1950.

Dean, P. The change from functional to primary nursing. *Nursing Clinics of North America,* 1979, *14*(2), 357–361.

De Brigard, P., & Helmer, O. *Some potential societal developments: 1970–2000.* Middletown, Conn.: Institute for the Future, 1970.

Delberg, P., & Van de Ven, A. A group process model for problem identification and program planning. *Journal of Applied Behavioral Science,* 1971, *7*(4), 466–491.

Dinkmeyer, D., & Carlson, J. *Consulting: Facilitating human potential and change processes.* Columbus: Charles Merrill, 1973.

Dinkmeyer, D., & Muro, G. *Group counseling theory and practice.* Atasca. Ill.: F. E. Peacock Publishers, 1979.

Egan, G. *Encounter: Group process or interpersonal growth.* Belmont, Calif.: Brooks/Cole, 1970.

Erickson, H., Tomlin, E., & Swain, M. *Modeling and role modeling.* Englewood Cliffs, N. J.: Prentice-Hall, 1983.

Erikson, K. *Human services today.* Reston, Va.: Reston Publishing Company, 1977.

Fitzgerald, L., & Murphy, J. *Quality circles.* San Diego: University Associates, 1982.

Gordon, T, et al. *The use of the Delphi technique in problems of educational innovation.* New York: Rand Corporation, 1976.

Green, T., & Petri, P. Nominal grouping: A theoretical model for organization effectiveness. In T. Green & D. Ray (Eds.), *Management in an age of rapid technology and social change.* Houston: Southern Management Proceedings, 1973, pp. 146–152.

Hodnett, E. *The art of working with people.* New York: Harper & Row, 1959.

Igoe, J. Project Health PACT in action. *American Journal of Nursing,* Nov. 1980, 2016–2021.

Jones, J. Dealing with disruptive persons in meetings. In J. Pfeiffer & J. Jones (Eds.), *The 1980 annual handbook for group facilitators.* San Diego: University Associates, 1980.

Koch, J. Use your nursing expertise in production manufacturing: Become a nurse consultant in industry, *Nursing '79,* July 1979, 72–73.

Kohnke, M. *The case for consultation in nursing.* New York: Wiley, 1978.

McCann-Flynn, J., Heffron, P. *Nursing from concept to practice.* Bowie, Md.: Robert J. Brady, 1984.

Pike, D. A practical approach to Delphi. *Futures,* 1970, *14*(2), 141.

Saunders, L., Chesley, D., & Kishi, A. Curriculum consultant, would you help us out? *Nursing and Health Care,* June 1981, 315–321.

Schutz, W. *FIRO: A three dimensional theory of interpersonal behavior.* New York: Rinehart, 1958.

Schwartz, A., & Goldiamond, I. *Social casework: A behavioral approach.* New York: Columbia University Press, 1975.

Shaw, M. *Group dynamics: The psychology of small group behavior.* New York: McGraw-Hill, 1976.

Shepherd, C. *Small groups.* Scranton, Pa.: Chandler, 1969.

Slack, P. School nursing in the USA: Aspect of clinical practice and managment. *Nursing Times,* March 13, 1980, pp. 468–469.

Smiley, O. The core committee: A model for decision-making within public health units. *Nursing Clinics of North America,* 1973, *8*(2), 355–358.

Tuckman, B. Developmental sequence in small groups. *Psychological Bulletin,* 1965, *63*(6), 384–389.

Tyler, R. *Basic principles of curriculum and instruction.* Chicago: The University of Chicago Press, 1969.

U. S. Department of Health and Human Services. *The school health curriculum project.* Atlanta: USDHHS, Public Health Service, Center for Disease Control, Bureau of Health Education; HHS publication number (CDC) 80-8359, 1977 (reprinted 1980).

Wilson, M. *Group theory/process for nursing practice.* Bowie, Md.: Brady Communications, 1985.

CHAPTER 10

The Nurse as Consultant to a Community

A community is like a ship; everyone ought to be prepared to take the helm.
Ibsen, An Enemy of the People, Act I

The group consulting relationships explored in Chapter 9 were those of primary groups. Cooley first used the term "primary group" in 1952 to define the smaller, personal-relationship groups characterized by intimate face-to-face associations in which members (other than the consultant) are usually already familiar with one another. But nurse consultants also work with community organizations and other large organizations referred to as secondary groups. Secondary groups are characterized as being larger, more diverse, and more impersonal in nature than primary groups. They present a different set of problems for the consultant. It is this type of secondary group relationship that is most prevalent in community consulting projects.

One form of community consultation frequently requested is for assistance in planning, organizing, developing, implementing, and evaluating the health services of multidisciplinary human service organizations. The range and diversity of these organizations are enormous. They include school systems, churches, medical centers, and the entire range of governmental health-funding agencies, community boards, and private foundations. Many viable health projects are conceived by these organizations in order to "help others," and most suffer from the lack of technical assistance at some point in time. Therefore, it is not unusual for community groups to seek help from professional paid or volunteer consultants with expertise in the particular area of need. Since many of these projects are health or screening clinics and involve direct service to consumers, the nurse is one of the most desired consultants to have on the consulting team.

In order to stress this type of community consultant activity, this chapter concentrates on two major areas: (1) an awareness of how community consultation differs in both theory and practice from either individual or small group consulting practice and (2) a case study of building a community primary health-care clinic.

The responsive and responsible consultant must realize that his or her role in community consultation is not just in changing individuals but in affecting whole communities. The kinds of services offered must be provided in accordance with the needs and wants of large numbers of clients and not always just in terms of traditional and comfortable nursing roles. Community consultation is both multifaceted and multidisciplinary in its approach. In community consultation, emphasis is on developmental and preventive approaches as well as on the remediation of existing problems. In this context, consultant function is aimed at helping the total community learn how to adapt, innovate, and plan on a continuous and orderly basis. In other words, the emphasis is on developing the capacity for self-renewal within individuals, subgroups, and the total community.

EARLY PHASES OF COMMUNITY CONSULTING

When a consultant is retained on a community project, it is frequently early on—that is, during the early planning stages before actual inception of the project itself. For example, when a community plans to build a health clinic, they frequently contract for the services of a consultant or a team of consultants to assist in planning, designing, and implementing the project. This early consultant input allows for more normal developmental sequences and for the prevention of problem areas. According to Morrill and associates (1974), the whole intent of engaging a consulting team is to anticipate future problems and move to prevent them by providing individuals or groups with needed skills, to create changes in the environment so as to prevent the development of problems, or at the least to keep a difficulty from becoming prevalent.

This emphasis on preventive consulting approaches, as contrasted with remedial approaches which deal with already existing problems or difficulties, will become more obvious in the case study of the development of a community health clinic presented later in this chapter. The general approaches to community consultation assume a much broader orientation than other forms of consultation, since they must (1) be aimed toward a large number of people, not just those who are experiencing some problem; and (2) be provided early, before some severe difficulty has already been identified.

A MULTISERVICE APPROACH

A nurse functioning as a community consultant will often discover that it is impossible to limit services to the solution of only nursing problems. There will undoubtedly be times that gaps in service delivery will exist and that the nurse consultant can only move toward greater effectiveness by recognizing commonalities with other helping professions, at times assuming their role and eliminating the tendency to see particular functions as "belonging to" one profession instead of another. For instance, if a community consulting team does not have a psychologist or social worker involved, the nurse may be the only one with the insight and skills in those professional areas to plan and design the roles for those professionals in the project. This does not imply that one specialist might replace another. Instead, it implies that the nurse consultant can recognize the need for other health disciplines and can ensure their inclusion in the final product.

Total team communication, collaboration, and cooperation are every bit as important as the coordination of diverse community groups. In fact, according to Bell and Nadler (1985), potential for dysfunctional conflict among team consultants is usually high, and its symptoms of ineffective communication and mutual antagonism are a definite hindrance to any project. The consulting team itself is an emerging small group, and effective team functioning calls for the same problem-solving methods and resolution of social conflict common to any group consulting process. Just as the core transaction of any consulting contract is the transfer of expertise from the consultant to the client, the core transaction of any consulting team is the transfer of expertise to the team member best prepared for the particular situation. This concept holds true whether the expertise is very tangible, such as skill in clinic design or nursing job descriptions, or very intangible, such as problem solving or team building.

Professional egoism is one of the most prevalent reasons for the breakdown of team cooperation. Consultants may fear the loss of individual prestige and worry that one's individual expertise will somehow get diluted and blurred. Thus, true collaboration is not an easy goal to attain and takes the effort and cooperation of each team member to achieve.

THE CONCEPT OF COMMUNITY

In the traditional sense of the concept, a community is a social group, territorially defined, that functions for the general welfare of its members (Lewis & Lewis, 1977). This functioning presupposes a commonality of attitudes and concerns and provides a basic unit for collective action. A community has social values, a social conscience, and common interests. It is concerned with the provision of services, including health care, for its members. Projects such as the establishment of a school health program or the planning of a primary health-care clinic can provide a common goal for community action. This common goal gives structure to a community group—structure that a nurse consultant must understand and deal with on an everyday basis.

But conversely, where there is a large secondary group united by a common goal, conflict also exists. Even small, fairly homogeneous communities evidence conflict and frequently are unable to function cooperatively enough to coordinate group action. As an example, later in this chapter a major case study of building a primary health-care clinic is presented that exhibits such varying degrees of conflict.

Much of the participation in organized health service programs is undoubtedly motivated by what psychologists call substitution or compensation for personal difficulties (Roemer, 1976). This is an important concept for the consultant to grasp. The consultant must be ready to handle conflict, since it invariably occurs in secondary group settings. This concept of conflict or resistance is so important that Gestalt psychologists, such as Lewin (1951), long ago identified it as a key concept in working with heterogeneous groups (Fig. 22), and Tuckman (1965) labeled it as the second stage (following orientation to the task) of task-activities development in his group process model (described in the "Group Function" section of Chapter 9).

Some additional early concepts of community conflict have been developed and published by Dahrendorf (1959). Even though Dahrendorf's work was focused on industrial communities, he spoke of a particular individual or interest subgroup as being the real agents of group conflict whenever interests are determined by a defined personal interest to the exclusion of the group as a whole or of what the community defines as the "common good." This type of conflict is ordinarily a political type of struggle and is characterized by defensiveness, competition, and jealousy. Political or power struggles tend to be the number one barrier or inhibitor to progress. They will, at times, block progress for weeks, and usually a whole series of internal modifications must subsequently take place before decision making and planned change can occur. This is probably the area of deepest concern for any community consultant, since the sense of failure can be overwhelming and a great deal of patience and tact is required during this period.

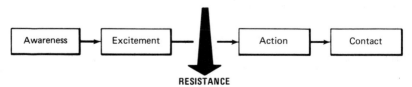

Figure 22. Resistances as conflict phenomena that occur between the excitement and action stages of the group decision-making process: A key concept of Gestalt psychology. *(From Lewin, K. Field theory in social science. New York: Harper & Row, 1951.)*

FROM CONCEPTS TO ACTION

The implementation of community consultation requires that the consultant exhibit some rather specific personal traits (Lewis & Lewis, 1977). These include the following:

1. An orientation toward being active instead of passive.
2. A sharp awareness of the social forces affecting individuals.
3. A willingness to take the risk of developing totally new techniques and skills.
4. An awareness that the nurse consultant is only one positive resource among many.
5. An ability to build new bases of support for a truly flexible approach.

To be flexible does not mean to lack guidelines for action but refers to a wide range of consultant activities carried out as an individual consultant, a team consultant, or a community liaison coordinator. For example, a nurse consultant under contract to a school system for the purpose of improving the school health education and school nursing program must engage in multiple community liaison activities—meeting with administrators, community leaders, teachers, parents, and students—in order to meet the needs of all school-age children. Cooperative planning and collaboration between the educational system and other community agencies are necessary to enhance the effectiveness of the school's total health program. Hence the consultant is involved during all stages and with all concerned agencies and groups in the affected communities. Only a program that will fulfill the health needs as identified by and in the community will be totally successful. Such consulting activities can be challenging and rewarding to the consultant as well as being a valuable contribution to the client system, the community as a whole.

The remainder of this chapter concentrates on an in-depth presentation of a sample case study emphasizing the consulting process and the nurse consultant's role in helping rural community members in their striving toward independence and effectiveness in building a much-needed clinic facility. The example presented could equally be applied to other consultant experiences in schools and organizations as well as to all voluntary or official health-care agency settings. The process, concepts, and principles remain the same regardless of the community setting.

A CASE STUDY OF COMMUNITY CONSULTATION: THE BIRTH OF AN IDEA

The major focus in this chapter is on the role of the nurse consultant as a member of a community consulting team involved in the planning, organization, development, implementation, and evaluation of a primary health-care clinic for a small rural community we will call Farmsville. The building of this clinic provides an exemplary case study of the community consulting process as it proceeds from entry to termination of the project.

The Farmsville community, a small southeastern rural town with a population of 704 persons, had recognized the need for local health-care services since Farmsville's last resident physician died 20 years ago. Repeated attempts to recruit physicians to practice in the area were unsuccessful, in part due to the fact that the physicians approached felt that as a single practitioner they would be swamped by demand. Other problems common to rural areas, such as the lack of social, recreational, and other fringe benefits that cities offer, also hindered physician recruitment.

However, at a Farmsville Town Council meeting, the council members were informed by a prominent leader in the community of the possibility of obtaining government help and funding to build a health clinic staffed by a nurse practitioner. As initiator of the project and first decision-maker, this influential woman continued to dominate the scene throughout the early phase of the project. With council agreement, she contacted the federal funding agency and, after an initial meeting with two staff members from the agency, scheduled an open meeting to be held in the Farmsville Town Hall. It was during this interim period before the meeting that the nurse consultant was approached by a staff representative of the federal agency and was invited to attend the meeting as a team member. A second consultant—an administrator with experience in clinical management—was also invited, as were interested representatives from concerned state and county agencies. This was the start of a nurse consultant relationship with a community group that had already identified as its primary goal the building of a health clinic in their town.

Stage One: Entry

First contact for a nurse consultant when dealing with community projects is usually through an intermediary agency, since such complex projects involve a number of individuals, groups, organizations, and interests both internal and external to the community. In this case study, the intermediary for the establishment of a rural primary health-care clinic—which are generally federally funded—was the regional health planning agency. Initially, the nurse consultant was selected as a result of networking—that is, a recommendation from an influential person familiar with the skills of the nurse as both practitioner and consultant. Thus the nurse as an expert in the area of concern joined a team formed to assist and guide the community's health planning board.

The first meeting held was an open community forum for the purpose of information exchange between consultants, the federal agency, community officials (mayor, fire chief, banker, and so on), the appointed temporary community health planning board, and interested citizens. In this setting the role of the nurse consultant was simply one of information-giver and professional expert, with emphasis on the discussion of the pros and cons of building a health-care facility in the community.

At this point, the climate of the community as a whole was receptive. Those attending were seeking information and help to solve an already identified problem. The climate was set for the beginning of a consultative relationship. The depth of underlying problems inherent in a group is difficult if not impossible to identify at this stage. The task of the consultant must be centered on the identification of norms or standards so that constructive interaction can take place during subsequent meetings.

The initial relationship of the nurse consultant to the community members and to the federal funding agency, and in turn their perception of the consultant as a helper and catalyst for change, was extremely important at this stage. The community was in the midst of a struggle to build a nurse practitioner clinic. Hence the nurse consultant's participation in the project was needed to meet the goals and objectives to be accomplished.

The need for the nurse consultant as a permanent member of the consulting team that would consist of the federal representative, the project administrator, and the nurse consultant was decided upon at the meeting, and tentative agreements were made to function as a team for the next six months. The funding for the clinic and for consultant contracts would come from federal grant monies. Thus the nurse consultant's role and responsibility in this setting was a dual one since there are two clients: (1) the federal planning agency and (2) the recipient of services, the community.

The first step, after the initial introductory phase, was to draw up a proposal describing the role of the nurse consultant for both the planning agency and the community. The fee schedule for the consultant as well as a tentative time allotment for the various stages of the project were also discussed and agreed upon. Figure 23 shows the proposal for nurse consultant activities.

Proposing a consulting plan of action is one of the first steps of contracting. The business of the contracting phase is to negotiate wants and needs, and to clarify all expectations on the part of both the consultant and client. In the case of community consultation, where so many different individuals and groups are involved, a written document describing the program and an explicit written agreement of what the consultant and client(s) expect from each other should be signed by both parties. A discussion of negotiating and contracting for consultant services, as well as a sample of a long-term contract, can be found in Chapter 12.

Even the earliest stages of a consulting project are not always free from group friction and high periods of emotional tension. As Tuckman (1965) pointed out, intragroup conflict typified by defensiveness, competition, and jealousy frequently causes a fight–flight period early in the relationship, as exemplified during the next (the second) community group meeting, which was designated for the purpose of electing board members.

The first task discussed at the meeting was the need to form a perma-

Subject: Proposal to function as a nurse consultant for the design and development of a rural nurse practitioner primary health-care clinic.

As a nurse consultant and a primary health-care nurse specialist, I am prepared to assist the planning agency staff and the community board to plan, develop, implement, and evaluate the following:

1. Identification of primary health-care service needs that a nurse consultant could fulfill
    1.1. Direction and guidance for assessing the health needs of a community service area
    1.2. Determine effectiveness of nursing services and nursing resources available
2. Design of a primary health-care program to meet community needs utilizing the nurse practitioner
    2.1. Determine nursing services to be provided
    2.2. Identify personnel requirements
    2.3. Write standards of nursing practice, job descriptions, and protocols to be followed
    2.4. Plan for record-keeping
    2.5. Plan for continuity of client care and setting up a referral system
    2.6. Set fee schedules for nursing service
3. Design the physical facility needs for an effective primary health-care clinic
    3.1. Evaluate the clinic site in view of its functional capacity
    3.2. Identify equipment, furniture, supplies, etc., that would be needed to maintain efficient function in a primary health-care clinic
4. Assist with the operational program
    4.1. Develop a contract and protocols for a physician preceptor, nurse practitioner, and nursing assistants
    4.2. Build in a program of continuing education for nursing personnel by providing a schedule of programs and liaison contact with nursing and health education departments of the state university for the first operational year
    4.3. Provide liaison for an ongoing evaluation of the effectiveness of the quality of the nursing care as well as the overall effectiveness of the primary health-care clinic

Figure 23. Sample proposal.

nent governing body of not less than nine nor more than 25 members. Specific guidelines for board membership were set forth in the federal grant guidelines:

> The majority of the board members will be persons who are or will be served by the project and who, as a group, represent the individuals being served, and no more than one-half of the remaining board members may be persons who derive more than ten percent of their income from the health-care industry. Employees of the project and their immediate families may not be board members, although project directors may serve as ex-officio, nonvoting members.

This statement of board composition was read at the meeting by the federal staff representative. Almost immediately there was a reaction from the group in the form of both awareness and objection to the fact that the prominent woman who had initiated interest in the clinic could not be a board member, since a member of her family would be the proposed nurse practitioner for the clinic. Arguments pro and con ensued and there appeared to be no satisfactory solution, until the nurse consultant—acting the role of arbitrator—pointed out that this person could serve as an ex-officio, nonvoting member of the board. This appeased the group and there was unanimous consent to appoint her to this position.

The information presented so far gives a background picture to the setting and identifies the overall goal for the consulting project, the building of a health clinic for the community. Additionally, during this first stage the need for certain assessment data was identified. For example, an earlier health survey of the area, documenting the existence of the need for a clinic, had to be reevaluated and updated. Thus the nurse consultant assumed another major role, moving from the role of expert and arbitrator to that of research director. A sample survey form was designed and volunteer members of the community conducted a door-to-door assessment under the supervision and guidance of the nurse consultant. The results more clearly defined the clinic's potential service population and gave a statistical determination of people in the area qualified for Medicare, Medicaid, or some form of insurance coverage. This was important knowledge for the future self-sufficiency of the clinic. Additionally, and throughout the entry stage, the nurse consultant's use of receiving as an intervention strategy played a decisive role in building acceptance, trust, and openness both in the relationships between the consultant and community leaders as well as between consultant and consulting team members.

Stage Two: Goal Setting
With the establishment of a functioning relationship between community and consultant, the Farmsville project moved into stage two, goal setting. At this point the role of the consultant team was to identify for the group problem areas that might be encountered in the future, and to assist the group in the identification of the tasks to be accomplished in order to build a health clinic (the primary goal). The delineation of major or secondary goals for steps such as obtaining legal counsel, deciding on building plans and site selection, and contracting for a physician preceptor, were generally agreed upon and then further broken down into subgoals (tasks) to be accomplished. As an example, three clear divisions for the construction of a clinic are apparent in this case study—that is, there would necessarily be an organizational or planning phase, a program development and building phase, and an actual opening or operational phase of the clinic. Subgoals for each of these three divisions would be developed jointly with the consulting team and the community group.

A sample list of identified goals for the consulting team and community to achieve during stage 2 is given in Figure 24. The list shown is by no means all-inclusive.

The importance of the guiding role of the nurse consultant as a team member during the goal-setting stage is apparent. The specific consultant

Organizational Subgoals

1. Increase community awareness of the health needs of the area and the need for a primary health-care clinic. Gain active and passive support from the total community
2. Establish a basic organizational structure with legal authority and responsibility so that subsequent activities can be carried out effectively
3. Conduct a health survey of the area in order to assess and document the existence of specific health problems and the need for a primary health-care clinic
4. Establish linkages and accumulate support for the clinic, and convert this support into an operational framework of cooperating agencies and health professionals
5. Develop an extramural proposal and submit the proposal to the proper agency for review

Program Development Subgoals

1. Enlist a representative group from the community that would form the permanent governing board and accept the responsibility for the ongoing supervision and continuing development of the clinic
2. Formalize the organizational framework by electing officers and appointing three committees to be responsible for: (a) articles of incorporation and by-laws, (b) site selection, and (c) personnel recruitment
3. Meet legal requirements through the filing of articles of incorporation as a nonprofit, private health organization
4. Interview and select the project administrator, the clinic receptionist–secretary, the nurse practitioner, and the physician sponsor (preceptor)
5. Reassess and document the existence of health problems and determine the primary care service area
6. Consolidate arrangements for health services to supplement those offered by the nursing clinic
7. Design a comprehensive program of primary health-care services to meet the present and future needs of the community
8. Determine the site for a physical plant for the clinic and secure an option for purchase or lease
9. Determine the architectural design, space requirements, and supply and equipment requirements for the clinic building
10. Prepare a detailed financial plan for program operation including operating costs, renovation costs, and anticipated revenue from the clinic
11. Design systems for billing, accounting, and patient record-keeping

Operational Phase Subgoals

1. Complete all plans for the opening of the clinic—that is, set opening date, etc.
2. Finalize all contracts with all clinic personnel plus auxiliary (part-time) personnel—dentist, mental health technician, social worker, physical therapist, and occupational therapist
3. Organize special community health programs with the physician sponsor and nurse practitioner as "public outreach" and clinic advertising
4. Finalize medical protocols, recording, and accounting systems

Figure 24. Sample goal list.

function is that of a transducer—a catalyst for planned change. Open communication at this point is vital. This communication process is not an easy task for the consultant with so many people involved. It requires intimate knowledge of all key community people. Certainly, the consultant must have already identified the community power structure, the outstanding decision makers and motivators (driving forces), as well as the passive members and the dissenters (restraining forces). Also, the consultant role moves rapidly during this stage from that of direct information-giver and clarifier of issues to facilitator and energizer.

This stage is characterized by numerous meetings with community group members and other health-care providers in which consultant activities are generally directed toward strengthening of group decisiveness and the formation of a coordinated nucleus of both community members and health-care providers. On occasion, it may be necessary to utilize confrontation as an intervention strategy, although this is a role more frequently found in the problem-solving and decision-making stages rather than in this overall goal-setting stage.

Stage Three: Problem Solving

Program development takes place during stage three, the problem-solving stage of the consulting process. Here the major role of the consultant turns to that of collaborator and gatekeeper, which primarily amounts to steering the client through the problem-solving process as well as supporting, facilitating, energizing, or confronting where needed. For example, when the community board involved itself in clinic site selection, a major conflict arose among the board members. Political factions and personal interests began to emerge. One member owned some land that she wanted to sell as a clinic site; the town banker had an interest in the renovation of an old theater which was the town "eyesore"; and another member wanted to rebuild the old train station. Tempers flared, and for a time there was real danger of the project being cancelled because of the strong emotional feelings and intractability of the individual members. The important role of the consultant here was to bring the group together (gatekeeper and facilitator), helping them keep on track and assisting them to come to some mutually acceptable decision. The conceptual model for analyzing alternate actions (see Fig. 16) was brought into play and provided the group with an effective decision-making tool that clearly identified a clinic site and still "saved face" for the dissenters. The use of a trailer as a clinic site was approved by all six board members. The table used for this analysis of alternate site selection is given as Figure 25.

The full participation of all concerned community members in this stage of problem solving must be emphasized. The consultant cannot become active in offering solutions or assuming responsibility for solutions. In fact, the expertise role of the consultant now transfers to the client group, which must now assume responsibility and direction of the project.

Possible Sites	Decision Criteria			
	Location—Accessible to Center Town	Parking Available	Renovation Cost	Rent and Reasonable Operating Costs
1. Old railroad station	Yes	Limited	High	Moderate
2. Vacated grocery store	Yes	No	Moderate	Low
3. Unoccupied highway cafe	No (3 miles)	Yes	Moderate	Low
4. Old theatre	Yes	No	High	High
5. Trailer on vacant lot	Yes	Yes	None (renovation money will buy trailer)	Low
Ideal solution (Trailer—#5)	Yes	Yes	Low	Low

Figure 25. Analyzing alternative actions in determining a clinic building site.

Also, it is not unusual that the problem-solving stage is marked by dissension culminating in power struggles between dominant personalities in the community, each vying for control. Even if tasks do get completed at this point, they often bear no relationship to the solidarity of the community group. The group will often appear confused and disorganized, which is usually exemplified by an impasse and inability to move into the decision-making stage. The role of consultant will also fluctuate to extremes, usually bringing into play all of the intervention strategies (as listed in Chapter 6) during this dissension phase. Remember that the group must work through its interpersonal problems before any constructive problem solving and progress can be made. "Face-saving" is important, and the consultant must be careful not to take sides but rather to take an objective and theoretical approach at this stage.

Stage Four: Decision Making

Stage four, the decision-making stage of the consulting process is one of client decision-making and client action, with the consultant now assuming the more passive role. Relying heavily on what has come before, it represents the focal point or main event of consultation. During this stage, the building of the clinic must take place and everything must fall neatly into place. Adversely, it is frequently the most trying stage for the consultant. It requires infinite patience and acceptance on the part of the consultant without being critical or condemning. It is a time for giving up the "reins" and leadership to the community group. The consultant role at this stage is much the role of an overseer, where the consultant stands at the sidelines and watches, ready at all times to assist the group to a more objective view of the situation where needed but letting the community representatives handle the problem or utilize existing resources to handle it wherever possible. There will be occasions when the community needs some help overcoming a limitation, but problem areas should be minimal during this stage.

The earlier use, in the problem-solving stage, of the conceptual model for analyzing alternative actions sets the stage for making sound, defensible judgments. Effective problem solving leads to decision making that is based on predictable consequences and that in turn forms the rationale or reasoning behind planned intervention. Coordination of activities of all the people involved in the development and building of the clinic would be the major work emphasis of the consultant during this period. The consultant cannot control all of the factors that occur unexpectedly and that may affect the ultimate development of the clinic, but if the preceding consultant interventions were effective, there will be a good outcome.

However, there may be times when even effective problem solving and planning do not lead to effective decision making. For example, even after the consultant's confrontation with the group over the site selection impasse, there were still dissident members of the community board who did not wholly accept what the group thought was their decision—the use of the trailer as a health clinic building. If this type of problem continues during the decision-making stage it calls for careful weighing of possible intervention strategies by the consultant. The problem may be that the consultant pushed the group too quickly to make a decision and that the group, or individual group members, did not have sufficient time to mull over the situation. Doing nothing until the group is ready to take a more objective view of the situation might be the intervention strategy of choice. On the other hand, lack of time might be a problem, and confrontation might again be the intervention strategy needed here.

Confrontation is not always a successful intervention and may even precipitate alienation between consultant and client. Like problem solving and the use of the model for analyzing alternative actions, confrontation is most effective when approached theoretically and objectively within a framework that clearly defines boundaries and can formulate a clear understanding of what happened as well as providing answers. The use of a modified nominal group process as defined in Chapter 9, and of the model for viewing and analyzing driving and restraining forces as presented in Chapter 7 (see Fig. 14), were the consultant's choices to serve this purpose. When applied to a decision-making impasse, such as in the problem of site selection, the following procedure is used:

1. State the general problem: "Members of the clinic board are still not in total agreement with the selection of a trailer for the health clinic."
2. Using the nominal group process, break the problem down into workable units. Have the group list all factors that influence the present situation. The list for this example is given in Figure 26.

The trailer lacks a feeling of permanance

It could be replaced by a more permanent building at a later date

It would not be on the main street of the town where it would have maximum visibility

It would be in close proximity to the main street (two town blocks)

There are perfectly good buildings in town that could be used

The trailer would contain more square footage than two of the other considered sites. Additional footage is not needed at this time

The trailer would be less costly to build and maintain than any other site considered

The trailer would contain all of the equipment and facilities needed for a health clinic at this time

Health clinics are not viewed by the public image as being in a trailer

Certain board members and other community leaders have personal interests in other proposed sites. The county owns the land proposed for the trailer, so this would not be a factor with the trailer as a site

Site selection has become a political as well as a personal profit motive

Figure 26. Factors influencing site selection.

By writing this breakdown of comments on a flipchart, the consultant was able to categorize them as a basis for group analysis and discussion. It was easy for the consultant to point out from the list that the group's responses moved from a subject-focused discussion of the use of a trailer as a clinic to the indirect psychological factors of personal and political interests.

The next step in getting around the impasse was to have the group view, sort, and list each factor as a positive (driving) force or as a negative (restraining) force for getting the clinic built. Forces could be labeled with a "D" (driving) or an "R" (restraining), or they could be separated into two columns. The latter technique is used in Table 10.

The point here is that problems are usually solved if they are approached systematically. Any effective methodology must be based on common sense. This use of the nominal group process and the viewing of the driving and restraining forces provided the group with the opportunity to clearly see that the negative factors were heavily weighted as inhibiting, interpersonal factors rather than being based on concrete thinking centered on building the clinic in the most feasible and realistic way. Furthermore, this particular approach to problem solving and decision making clarifies for the group certain concepts that may have previously been on an unconscious level, and enables the group to analyze the forces one by one and identify individual strategies for dealing with each.

However, there may be times when an open nominal group discussion only increases the group's already high anxiety level; the approach presented above then may not be the process of choice for the situation. In such instances, it would be better for the consultant to consider the use of the

TABLE 10. FACTORS AFFECTING USE OF TRAILER AS CLINIC

Positive (Driving Forces)	Negative (Restraining Forces)
1. It could be replaced at a later date	1. Lacks feeling of permanance
2. It is within two blocks of the center of town	2. It is not in the center of town
3. It has adequate square footage	3. There are other good buildings that could be used
4. It would be less costly to build and maintain than any other proposed site	4. A trailer does not portray the public image of a health clinic
5. Could contain all equipment and facilities needed at this time	5. People have personal interests in other sites
6. Land costs not politically or profit oriented	6. Other sites involve political as well as personal interests

more impersonal mail-in Delphi technique (described in Chapter 9) for gathering data before calling a meeting.

Finally, during this stage it is important that the consultant assist the community group to take an evaluative look at how each task was accomplished or why it was not accomplished. As Blake and Mouton (1983) remarked, a good consultant teaches theory to clients, who in turn use such systematic insights to phase out of their own self-defeating cycles. In other words, a client should be aided through theory-based consultant interventions to comprehend what causes things to be as they are, to predict consequences that can be expected, and to be able to shift the cause and effect variables operating in the situation.

Stage Five: Termination

Planning, building, and operating a community primary health-care clinic is a long-range project. As such, disengagement is also a long-term, gradual process so that continuity and the continuing development of the project are ensured. Thus in stage five, termination, contracts may need to be renegotiated so that the community has access to the expertise, reinforcement, and encouragement that is certain to be needed in the future. The big questions of termination are how much, how fast, and how soon?

The consultant must always remember that a goal of consulting is to teach clients how to solve similar problems in the future. If the consultant plans to work with the community after the immediate project is completed, then there should be a clear understanding of what to expect. The consultant role should again be that of expert advisor, with the community accepting the day-to-day responsibility for clinic function. This does not rule out the possibility of reactivation to a more active consulting role if the need again arises.

It is difficult to withdraw from a successful project just as it is all too easy to want to avoid a project when it isn't going well. This factor was all too evident in the case study presented in this chapter. The original six-month contractual agreement was renegotiated three times and continued for a total period of 14 months. Even then, it was the nurse consultant rather than the community that had to make the decision for final termination, and then only after an agreement that the community board could call for additional services if the need again surfaced. It never did, because the disengagement was a gradual process and characterized by a period of testing—determining whether or not the community was able to function independently in the new clinic situation.

Also during disengagement the process of evaluation should be very evident, and when the time for closure arrives it should be distinguished by both the community and the consultant acknowledging that they are now moving into this final phase. One contribution that the consultant can make at the end of a project is to point out to the client what they did well. The client should also provide feedback to the consultant so that the final evaluation is a mutual process. Closure should not be viewed as a rejection of the consultant, but rather as a signal of the successful completion of a particular assignment and relationship.

In conclusion, the termination stage in a long-range community project is usually characterized by the following features:

1. Gradual reduced involvement by the consultant and an assuming of responsibility by the community group.
2. Involvement does not generally drop to zero but may continue at a very low level, drawing on the consultant more for advice, expertise, and encouragement than for active participation.
3. Termination even when completed leaves the door always open for further work with the community as needed.

SUMMARY

Many other examples of community consultation could have been included in this chapter. But most would be similar in their activities and in the types of problems presented. Specific skills and techniques are the same and only the setting changes. Large secondary groups present diverse consulting problems. Stage 1, entry, is particularly important, since it takes a lot more time and experience to form meaningful working relationships between the consultant and such a large client system.

A formal written contract is a must in community consultation because of the complexity of the situation. Verbal agreements are not adequate protection for consultant or community. Also, the community size and diversity of interests frequently cause problems of group dissension, resulting in power struggles between dominating personalities vying for political control, and with the consultant caught in the middle.

From the case study presented in this chapter it is apparent that problem solving in large groups is too complex and flexible to be reduced to an exact pattern. In theory, according to Hodnett (1959) in *The Art of Working with People,* something like the following should and often does happen:

1. Diagnosis
   a. Examine the general problem situation for background
   b. Identify and state the problem
   c. Analyze the problem
   d. Establish criteria for judging solutions
   e. Set up guidelines for procedure
2. Attack
   a. Isolate the most logical areas of concentration
   b. Offer ideas freely, both hypothetical and practical
   c. Feed back alternative solutions
   d. Estimate their validity
   e. Determine areas for further exploration
   f. Offer further alternatives
   g. Feed back what has been achieved
3. Decision making
   a. Make decision, repeat procedure, or restructure the problem
   b. Test preferred solution
   c. Recommend and initiate action

Community consultation presents a major challenge for any consultant. The role the consultant plays will fluctuate to extremes in such a complex situation and all consultant skills and intervention strategies come into play in order to facilitate the group decision-making process. The application of a strong theoretical framework is of vital importance to the successful completion of the consulting relationship.

Finally, most community projects do not terminate consultant intervention suddenly. Rather, the final stage is more a process of gradual disengagement and ongoing evaluation before final closure is obtained.

SELECTED REFERENCES

Bell, C., & Nadler, L. *Clients and consultants.* Houston: Gulf Publishing Company, 1985.

Blake, R., & Mouton, J. *Consultation* (2nd ed.). Reading, Mass.: Addison-Wesley, 1983.

Brown, E. *Nursing reconsidered: A study of change—The professional role in community nursing.* Philadelphia: Lippincott, 1971.

Cohen, M. Citizen participation in the decision-making activities of formal social service agencies: An unreasonable goal? *Community Mental Health Journal,* 1976, *12*(4), 355–363.

Dahrendorf, R. *Class and class conflict in industrial society.* Stanford: Stanford University Press, 1959.

Gallessich, J. Organizational factors influencing consultation in schools. *Journal of School Psychology,* 1973, *11*(1), 57–65.

Hodnett, E. *The art of working with people.* New York: Harper & Row, 1959.

Lange, F. *The design and development of a rural nurse practitioner primary health care clinic: A study of the decision-making process with emphasis on the role of the nurse consultant.* An Unpublished doctoral dissertation. The University of Alabama in Birmingham, 1979.

Lewin, K. *Field theory in social science.* New York: Harper & Row, 1951.

Lewis, J., & Lewis, M. *Community counseling: A human services approach.* New York: Wiley, 1977.

Morrill, W., Oetting, R., & Hurst, J. Dimensions of counselor functioning. *Personnel and Guidance Journal,* 1974, *56*(6), 354–359.

Roemer, M. *Rural health care.* St. Louis: The C.V. Mosby, 1976.

Tuckman, B. Developmental sequence in small groups, *Psychological Bulletin,* 1965, *63*(6), 384–399.

PART IV

Issues in Consultation

Part IV focuses on two phenomena that are an integral part of the everyday experiences encountered by the practicing consultant: (1) the ethical issues that pertain to human relations consulting and (2) the business issues of marketing, negotiating, and contracting.

Unlike nursing, consultation has yet to achieve the kind of professional stature that is accompanied by enforceable codes of conduct. Nevertheless, every nurse consultant is confronted with issues of fairness, honesty, and effectiveness. The list of issues that can fall on a right–wrong continuum are numerous. A number of these issues are identified and examined in Chapter 11. These issues constitute some of the major problem areas that consultants must consider during any consulting relationship.

Chapter 12 moves into the area of nurse entrepreneurship and details the marketing, negotiating, and contracting techniques that are so vital to a successful consulting experience for both consultant and client. One of the most critical skills in consultation is to put into words what the client wants from the consultant and what support the consultant can expect from the client. The importance of establishing sound positive professional relationships across the areas of marketing, negotiating, and contracting cannot be overemphasized. Without exception, all of the misunderstandings and distrust that can occur in a consulting relationship can be avoided by having an explicit contractual agreement. Sample short and long-form contracts are included in this chapter. Also included in Chapter 12 are many of the business techniques and detailed administrative factors involved with providing consultant services. This chapter provides important information and guidelines for nurse consultants regardless of their part-time or full-time status or internal versus external consultant classification.

Consultant planning and efficient management of the everyday activities of consulting are critically important for success. This book has a practical emphasis and contains multiple consulting techniques and applications, but it must all be put together in some consecutive order to be effective. This ordering of the essential steps and consultant tasks comprises the final chapter of this book, Chapter 13. It is here that the total consulting process is put together and defined using a checklist format. This checklist provides a handy reference for the practicing nurse consultant.

CHAPTER 11
Ethical Issues in Consulting

The unique aspect of man is that he communicates with his fellow man through speech, amulets, laws, and codes of ethics. . . .

G. Lippitt, 1973, p. 7

Like any other profession, as the field of nursing consultation grows it becomes more important than ever to face the questions of ethical behavior in consulting practice. With increased growth, the probability of questionable activities related to ethics, legalities, and values is increased. Consequently, when some members of the profession are seen to act in less desirable ways, the entire profession loses. For this reason, as a profession matures, codes of ethics are usually created for the group. Consultation, at the present time, has not formulated its specific code for consultant behavior but rather depends on the ethical code in the consultant's own professional field to serve this purpose.

ETHICS

Ethics are the codes or standards of conduct based upon consensus values that have already been set (Hansen et al., 1972). Ethics then, as viewed by such authors as Curtis and Flaherty (1982), Davis and Aroskar (1983), Donnelly and associates (1980), and Taylor (1975), are a system of valued behaviors and beliefs, and as such represent a personal, professional, or institutional code of behavior that depends a great deal on beliefs about humanity, right and wrong, and good and evil. However, rightness and wrongness are not always mutually exclusive. What one person, profession, or institution perceives as right may be viewed as wrong by another.

A good example of this are the variations in the standards, values, and orientations held by different individuals in the United States on the question of legalized abortion. Just as in the abortion situation, it seems impossible to avoid the impingement of personal values in consulting. Each consultant has identifiable values, whether presented covertly or overtly. The client also has values and value dilemmas. The main task of the consultant is not to transmit what he or she considers to be the "right" ethical values, but to help clients clarify their own position so that they can identify the values that best suit the situation.

When ethics are viewed as statements of what should be and not what is, it becomes easier for the consultant to utilize ethical codes as a point of reflection and comparison for the conduct of service during the consulting relationship. According to Fenner (1980), ethical standards are closely correlated with personal value systems. Introspection and analysis of personal values and interpretation of value systems in view of professional ethics allows the consultant to develop the skills necessary for ethical consulting practice without nonconformity with personal standards.

NORMS AND VALUES

As Lippitt (1973) pointed out, a professional system such as consulting will develop expected and prescribed ways of acting in relationship to its goals and objectives. For the nurse consultant, these standards of behavior will be dually influenced by the nursing profession as well as by past experiences in consulting. For example, in nursing these norms will include how the nurse dresses in a hospital setting, in a public health setting, or when working as a consultant. Many such norms are powerful dictums. In consultation, to act contrary to the norms may bring severe censorship or even total rejection by the client. Consultation, like all other social systems, must develop a system of expected behavior that determines the interrelationships between consultant and client and, thereby, the whole structure of consultation.

Values and ethics go hand in hand. While ethics refer to a general or professional code of behavior, and values are more concerned with the relative worth, merit, or usefulness of an ideal or principle, each is part of the other. This relationship of human interaction is demonstrated in Figure 27 as an exchange communication of ethics and values between consultant and client. Occasionally there is reluctance or neglect on the part of a consultant to identify and consider the personal and professional value systems that guide his or her interventions. Yet the process of value information and clarification is all-important to the consulting relationship. Every consultant intervention includes a decision based on values and goals as a

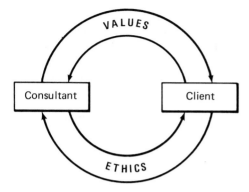

Figure 27. The exchange communication of values and ethics.

part of the two-way dialogue that occurs between consultant and client. Identifying one's own value system and helping clients review, clarify, and confront their values and goals may be one of the most important measures that the consultant can offer.

VALUE CLARIFICATION

Warwick and Kelman (1976) define values as individual or shared conceptions of the desirable—that is, "goods" considered worth pursuing. Since values determine the choice of goals toward which change effort is directed, it is important that the consultant have a clear perception of how the client comes to hold certain beliefs and establish certain behavior patterns.

Values are such an intrinsic part of a person's life experiences that it is impossible to trace their origins or even to examine them rationally. There are some things that are valued in themselves. To the majority of the people in the United States, marriage and children are such values. Other things are valued because of their consequences or effects but not in themselves; it is a good thing to go to a dentist even though it can be a traumatic experience. The value is in wanting healthy teeth and the act of visiting the dentist is valued not as an end in itself but as a means to a goal.

In the practical affairs of everyday life, people hold many such values, but do not stop to make detailed calculations every time they choose a course of action. Choices are made on the basis of common sense and because of similar situations faced in the past. In most valuing situations, the individual uses only reasoning and imagination to make a reasonable prediction about what would happen as the result of such an act (Taylor, 1975).

The consultant's role lies beyond the realm of the client's everyday value judgments. Rather, it is concerned with the process of value clarification whenever controversial issues arise that the client cannot handle alone. Values clarification is the process of assessing, exploring, and determining what these personal values are and what priority they hold in the client's decision-making process (Fenner, 1980). Value clarification focuses on helping the client to develop skills in formulating judgments and making choices of his or her own in four areas: cognitive (thinking), affective (feeling), active (helping), and interpersonal (communicating).

Furthermore, the valuing process according to Simon (1971) is composed of seven subprocesses:

1. Helping each individual to make free choices when possible.
2. Searching for alternatives in choice-making situations.
3. Analyzing the consequences of each alternative.
4. Considering what each person prizes and cherishes.
5. Publicly affirming the things that each individual values.
6. Doing something or acting on the choices available.
7. Identifying and strengthening the positive patterns in each individual's life.

An important by-product of helping the client to define and clarify values is the learning process that occurs, thereby enabling the client to apply value clarification principles to the solution of problems in the future.

CONFLICTING VALUES

A real problem arises when conflicting values between consultant and client emerge. Such conflicts are bound to arise during the course of consulting relationships. As Donnelly and associates (1980) note in *The Nursing System: Issues, Ethics, and Politics,* serious conflicts do not "go away" if they are ignored and unresolved. Rather, suppressed or unresolved conflicts lead to interpersonal hostility and task disruptions that keep the system unbalanced. A consultant must not retreat from conflict but should use it as a challenge to develop new skills in communicating and collaborating. Thus, conflict is not always bad: it can be a stimulus for the consultant to examine his or her own ethical values and perspectives and develop new and better approaches.

There are occasions during conflict when the problems between consultant and client cannot be readily solved. If such is the case, it may be necessary for the consultant to confront the client in order to discuss openly the discrepancies that may be occurring between words and actions. Confrontation can take different methods of attack. For example, a particular faculty group may have agreed to participate in a group project to revise curriculum but failed to carry out agreed-on tasks. Possible reasons for this discrepancy should be discussed. The consultant might begin by stating:

> You say that you are interested in changing the curriculum, yet you have not completed the last two assignments that we agreed on. Let's take a look and make sure that we both understand what was to be done and why and how we could make it easier to carry out.

If this exploration yields no explanations, the consultant may remind the group about the agreement, pointing out that it is a waste of both consultant and group time, effort, and money if they do not shoulder the responsibility for achieving outcomes. In this kind of a situation, the consultant needs to be firm and supportive at the same time. If concord cannot be reached, perhaps the overall consulting contract will have to be reassessed. This example lends itself to a relatively simple consultant confrontation intervention.

On the other hand, during the community consulting experience cited in Chapter 10, the consultant assisting a rural group in the development of a nursing clinic ran into a seemingly insurmountable dispute among members of the client group regarding the location of the clinic. Three members of the group had their own ideas and personal reasons for proposing different locations, and no one would back down because they felt that their own value systems and personal integrity were being challenged by both the group and the consultant. This controversy over what should have been an easy decision to make, exemplifies the power that value conflict can have on a group or even a total community. It took consultant confrontation intervention of "either you select the site or I dissolve the contract" to break the deadlock. The end result was a compromise on site selection. Maybe not the best site, but at least a solution that was necessary for problem solving, decision making, and project progression.

Throughout any value clarification process, the client must be actively involved. The consultant approach is to assist the client to use creative ability in order to facilitate clarification and subsequent decision making. However, when conflicting values do occur, confronting statements may have to be made by the consultant in order to help clients become more aware of what they are or are not doing.

ETHICAL DECISION MAKING

The exploration of values calls for the same decision-making approach that the consultant uses to assist the client in exploring alternative actions and weighing the probability, value, and risk of the outcomes (see Chapter 7 for a discussion and models of problem solving and decision making). This approach to analysis is a very useful one whenever it is the client's own value system, not the consultant's, that enters into the decision. The consultant, in most ethical decision making, is not making a decision about consultant activities but rather is helping and facilitating client decision making. In this type of situation, remember that the problem is the client's problem. Therefore, the problem of which alternative to choose is the client's prerogative. The consultant's problem is how to help the client in the process of decision making.

Moreover, it is important that the consultant be aware of and able to resolve the ethical problems associated with the practice of consultation. Clearly ethical issues, falling in the realm of consulting practice, are often intertwined with both conceptual and factual (empirical) issues. To pick a fairly simple example, suppose the consultant is concerned with the theoretical acceptability of a particular nursing home that is the choice of a family for an invalid mother. The consultant, on the other hand, has heard many undocumented instances whereby this particular home does not meet the standards of quality that it should. In this situation, the consultant's basic concern is with the issue of acceptable placement and care to the satisfaction of the family. This is their choice. However, the consultant must face the problem of his or her own value clarification on the nature of the issue. This is a case of ethical theory as applied in the light of conceptual structures and the factual (actual) beliefs of the consultant. Consequences to the client are all-important here.

What, then, is the consultant's responsibility? Does this come under the category of withholding information from the client? If yes, then under what conditions is this justified? "An ethical theory provides a set of moral principles which is to be used in assessing what is morally right and what is morally wrong with regard to human action" (Mapes & Zembaty, 1980, p. 4). But in the situation of the nursing home, where evidence is heresay, there is no right or wrong. Perhaps the consultant's "most fundamental right" is the right to self-determination. The consultant's determination of the information that the client needs to have in order to make a rational decision, and then letting the client make the decision, comprise ethical decision making.

CONFIDENTIALITY

Maintaining confidentiality is a common problem in both nursing and consulting and is a major area of ethical behavior facing the nurse consultant. Confidentiality involves the retention of information received in a personal interaction with the client. Sometimes the information or data considered confidential cannot be treated as completely confidential. For example, Hansen and associates (1972) see confidential information as existing at several levels, as follows:

1. *The first level* is professional use of information. Here, whatever discussion occurs other than with the client is done professionally with those who have a degree of understanding as to the meaning of the information. This information is released with the client's consent. Such information would be related to technical documents, records, and other data that might exist about and outside the client.
2. *The second level* involves information that is transmitted from the client on a personal basis during the consulting interview. A plan of

handling such confidential material should have been clarified early in the consulting relationship. Certainly the client should be informed of the consultant's intentions to utilize this personal information.

3. *The third level* of confidentiality is that the consultant simply does not divulge any material given by the client. Two exceptions here would be if clear danger to human life exists or if the client consents to divulging the information.

Sometimes honoring professional confidences may lead to awkward predicaments. This problem arises most commonly when an inquirer approaches the consultant seeking information about the client but the inquirer's authority to receive such information cannot be verified. Also, through careless talk in a public place confidential information may inadvertently be revealed to persons who should not have access to it. A pertinent question related to confidentiality posed by French (1974) is "where does professional interest in the scientific elements of the case end and violation of confidence begin?" (p. 90).

Violating confidentiality is an obvious moral or ethical breach. Yet the problem is compounded for the consultant, since access to people and information are the key requirements of any consultant. Information not only about technical data but also regarding the attitudes of the client and others toward the problem, as well as information about their roles and responsibilities, is needed for effective consultant intervention. Hence the consultant is intimately involved with the personal confidences of others. Very often, the consultant is caught in the "trap" of not being able to perform effectively because of ethical confidentiality. Perhaps the best approach is to give clients control of identifying people they wish to involve in the relationship or to share the findings with. This gives the clients a choice about how to protect themselves, if necessary.

OTHER ETHICAL CONSIDERATIONS

Ethical conflicts arise because of the relationship of some event to the existing value system of either the consultant or the client. In citing another example, there are times when the consultant may face an ethical conflict when the client decides to do something dishonest.

When terminating a consulting project with a director of nursing, the director demands that a statement be put into the consultant's report placing blame for a poor job of planning staffing needs onto a particular nursing supervisor. The consultant knows for a fact that the nursing supervisor was overruled in her design of the original staffing plan by the nursing director, and made to change and lower standards. Thus, unwarranted blame is to be placed on the wrong person and the supervisor would certainly be injured (if not professionally, at least personally) by such a report. In this case, the consultant has an ethical obligation to refuse to write such a report and even to cancel the contractual agreement at this late date if the nursing director refuses to cooperate.

At other times in another situation, such blame placed on a third party may be factual, leaving the consultant with yet another dilemma—that of weighing with the client the consequences of such an accusation on the entire consulting project.

There are many such specific areas of ethical behavior facing the nurse consultant. The remainder of this chapter discusses nine issues that pertain to human relations consulting. These issues are not inclusive—that is, there may be other identifiable issues. However, these nine are viewed by the author as the more common issues affecting consultant behavior. Some are clearly questions of ethics. Other topics do not fit into the ethical–unethical category but rather concern themselves with the responsibilities of prudent, competent, professional consultants. It should also be noted that the issues are alphabetized rather than prioritized since no one issue is of greater importance than the other.

Accountability

Consultants must always remain aware that they are accountable. In the first place, the consultant is accountable for examining self-motivations, the results desired, and the methods employed. Secondly, the consultant must identify how well these things consistently correspond with the value responses required of him or her as a professional. The consultant is also accountable to the client and all those affected in the interchange.

Accountability holds the consultant answerable for the extent to which actions taken are consistent with the consultant's responsibility. The area of accountability includes awareness of self-limitations. As a case in point, a major ethical issue of accountability relates to the presentation of the consultant's professional qualifications. If a consultant is inaccurately represented by someone as having extensive experience in a particular area, it is the responsibility of the consultant to correct the misrepresentation. Not all consultants, even in the same discipline, are equally expert or competent in dealing with a particular range of problems that may present themselves in a consulting situation. The consultant is responsible for defining self-limitations of skill, knowledge, and expertise.

The consultant who does not define what is reasonably possible in a given period of time, with the resources and limits at hand including self-limitations, usually tries to do too much or tries to cover all the bases too quickly. This leads to disillusionment and often to frustration and failure. Only when contractual agreements are defined as to what can reasonably be expected can things be done in a rational way (Schulberg & Killilea, 1982). The consultant has an ethical responsibility to clear up all actual or implied inaccuracies of qualifications, experience, and education.

Another aspect of the consultant's responsibility to the client is evaluated by examining the actual performance in relation to the expected performance. Here quality assurance is the term used to denote structure and process involved in assuring that the client receives the type of consultation activity advantageous to the attainment of the goal. Quality assurance, as described by Patton (1980), involves consultant introspection in:

1. Evaluating the excellence of results derived from the consulting relationship.
2. Taking actions to make improvements that are likely to affect a higher quality of consultative activities in the future.

The final consideration under accountability is the need for the consultant to become knowledgeable about the ethical standards most closely related to his or her professional description and consulting position. The nurse consultant should know not only the ethical standards of professional nursing but also those professional standards more closely related to consulting and counseling. The American Personnel and Guidance Association is one organization that publishes such standards.

Authority

Conflicting authority and power have been previously discussed, but are important enough to warrant reemphasis. Both authority and power have the ability to cause and prevent change. The simple fact of being hired to do a job gives the consultant the authority to act in a consulting situation. However, power must be shared by both the consultant and the client, and the task to be accomplished must be agreed upon by both.

Authority, by definition (Stein & Su, 1980), is the power to act, judge, or command—that is, to carry out the responsibility assigned or assumed by the consultant. Authority, then, is a necessary condition for the effective achievement of consultant–client goals. The differentiation between authority and power is that authority usually refers to legitimized power, the right to function in a particular role; while power, which is the potential of one person to have an effect on the attitudes, perceptions, and behavior of another, can be used effectively or misused.

Thus the common factor in authority is power. Clients as well as consultants have the potential for the exercise of power. Power elements appear to be present in all forms of consultation. The key to effective consultation lies in the open acknowledgment of this power by both consultant and client. This open acknowledgment, according to Langford (1981), holds the greatest promise for maximizing objective problem solving. Consultation is not a unidirectional authority–power process. In fact, the same processes that act to foster consultant power also act to foster client power. Power is only effective when balanced by a feeling of commonality that leads to a genuine liking and respect on the part of both consultant and client.

Autonomy

Autonomy is the freedom of decision making and the right to determine one's own acts. It enables the consultant to initiate the type and depth of intervention that will be most effective. Certainly the consultant has autonomy; yet autonomy, like accountability, has boundaries that can produce problems as well as privileges. Pfeiffer and Jones (1977) point out that autonomy of the consultant arises from three main sources:

1. Specialized knowledge required to practice as a consultant.
2. Need on the part of the consultant to provide a necessary and valuable service to the client.
3. The client. Clients grant a consultant autonomy on the basis of a "trust" that the consultant will place concern for the client above self-concern.

Additionally, autonomy is influenced by the values and ethics of the professional group (nursing), by the laws governing the profession, and by guidelines initiated by peers (Donnelly et al., 1980). The autonomy of the consultant does not permit the consultant to force any private ethical views or values on the client even if they are in harmony with the client's values and goals. Autonomy demands that both consultant and client choose their moral principles independently of external constraints. In fact, the task of the consultant is not only autonomy in consulting activities but also the fostering of autonomous decision making and action in the client. Robert Wolff (1976) defines the autonomous person as follows:

> The autonomous man, insofar as he is autonomous, is not subject to the will of another. He may do what another tells him, but not because he has been told to do it. . . . For the autonomous man, there is no such thing, strictly speaking, as a command. (p. 14)

Both the autonomous consultant and the autonomous client have the ability to step back and formulate an attitude toward the factors that influence their behavior.

Coercion

Coercion is the misuse of power, and takes place when a consultant forces a client into doing something he or she really does not want to do. Warwick and Kelman (1976) found that coercion basically arises in two circumstances:

1. A client wants to perform a certain action, or in the normal course of events would perform this action, but is constrained from doing so by physical means or the threat of severe deprivation by the consultant.
2. Alternatively, a client desires not to perform a certain action or normally would not carry out this action, but actually does so because of physical compulsion or threats by the consultant.

Conversely, coercion can be a client behavior, wherein the consultant may be threatened with the loss of a job if client demands are not acquiesed to in a particular situation. It is difficult to arrive at a precise definition of "threat" or "deprivation," but they refer to the loss of something that is highly valued. In a consulting relationship the threat that the client will not reach a goal and will therefore be a failure is frequently enough pressure and coercion to make the client change a decision or action. Coercion should also be distinguished from compliance occurring within the framework of legitimate authority. Compliance is conformity to behave in a particular manner. For example, compliance with the traffic laws is necessary for safe driving. In a sense this could be viewed as a type of coercion, but in compliance people act in the belief that it is right to do so. This belief of "right" is not present in coercion.

Coercion is almost never ethically justified in a consulting relationship, especially if there is no great threat to basic societal values. There may occasionally be the need for prompt and positive action to accomplish the goals of the consulting project, but even in such a situation an ethical justification of coercion requires the consultant to demonstrate, rather than assume, the threat to basic values. The legal concept of "clear and present danger" would seem to be an appropriate test of any proposal for coercion, and the defense of coercion usually rests on personal evaluations of the system in question (Warwick & Kelman, 1976). The consultant should protect the right of the client to refuse participation in any activity as desired. For example, in a workshop or in-service education program, the participants should not be coerced by the consultant to participate in any activity when they show a reluctance to do so. It is unethical to force people in a group situation to participate against their wishes. If the consultant pressures the person or the group, it could create unnecessary anxiety. Pfeiffer and Jones (1977) stress the fact that the consultant must be sensitive to the emotions, feelings, beliefs, values, and wants of the clients and not use methods that deviate markedly from participants' behavior expectations.

Fee Setting

In consultation what is being sold is the consultant's capability or service for a certain time under certain conditions. The product of the consultant's labor, or the benefit of the consultant's services, then belongs as property to the client. The question of selling consulting services for a fee is an ethical question, since a free market exists in consultation and fee setting is a matter of individual consultant prudence. Thus, unethical fee setting, or overcharging, is an issue that each consultant must deal with. The consultant who knowingly becomes involved in such an unethical practice negates professional responsibility for personal gain and jeopardizes the public confidence and trust in both the consulting and nursing professions. Under the American Nurses' Association (ANA) *Code for Nurses* (1976) such unethical behavior as false advertising (fee setting is a part of this code structure) may result in the reprimand, censure, suspension, or expulsion of the nurse from the association for violations of the code.

Pfeiffer and Jones (1977) point out several potential issues regarding consulting fees. First, it seems to be a fairly common practice for consultants to vary the amount they charge according to their client's ability to pay. Another issue is the opportunity of the consultant to pad an expense account or charge the client for either time or materials not delivered. There is also the issue of submitting additional bills after the client has already paid what they considered the final bill.

It is the responsibility of the consultant to ensure that the fee agreement with the client is written into the contract and is explicit in terms of cost and agreed-upon expenses. It is not unprofessional to discuss financial arrangements. It is not necessary to belabor the financial aspect, but to ignore it is to court financial disaster. The consultant must take responsibility for fee setting either hourly, daily, or by the case. It is unrealistic to assume that the client will understand consulting practice and make a financial offer. Consultants should know their own "worth" and be familiar with competitive rates within the field (for more specific details see the "Fee Setting" section of Chapter 12).

Manipulation

One of the frequent ethical problems involved with consultation is the question of whether or not it is appropriate for the consultant to plan interventions for clients without their consent or participation in the planning. This is generally considered manipulation, which is defined by Warwick and Kelman (1976) as "a deliberate act of changing either the structure or alternatives in the environment (environmental manipulation) or personal qualities affecting choice without the knowledge of the person involved (psychic manipulation)" (p. 486).

No physical compulsion or threats of deprivation are involved in manipulation as they are in coercion. Rather, the cardinal feature of this process is that it maintains the semblance of freedom while modifying the framework within which changes are made. This type of manipulation is so common that there may be times when even the consultant is not aware that he or she is doing the manipulating. There are even times when it can be a necessary and desirable activity. Perhaps the key question is how far manipulation goes and to what end the client is being controlled. These are value judgments and, from an ethical standpoint, the principle difference lies in the degree to which the individuals affected may control the process.

Privacy

There is considerable concern today about the invasion of privacy by the helping professions. Privacy has already been touched on under the other headings, but so far attention has been focused upon the information level rather than physical invasion of privacy.

All too frequently the consultant "pushes" to work and achieve far beyond the client's physical or even desired mental capabilities. This tendency for the consultant to get the work done in as short a time as possible can result in physical and mental harrassment of the client. Too frequent telephone calls, interrupting the client with unannounced visits, and generally "crowding" the client are examples of interference with the client's right to privacy.

The consultant's responsibility is to protect the client's privacy, not to abuse it. Greater care must be taken to ensure that the privacy of the client and significant others is maintained. What is advocated here is that the consultant accept the client's felt needs to work at a pace compatible with a level at which the client can serve as a competent and willing collaborator.

Sexuality

Sexuality in the nurse consultant role presents many of the same problems faced every day in the nursing role. Whenever the consultant role is used to establish sexual relations with a client or other project participant, the consultant has clearly violated the standards of ethical behavior.

Often as the consulting relationship grows, the bonds of trust and feelings of mutual affection also develop. This issue of growing affection is somewhat complicated. Such affection can make the relationship pleasant and facilitate growth; on the other hand, it can create problems for the consultant, especially when the client's expressions of affection impinge on the limits of a professional helping relationship (Sundeen et al., 1981). Also, the consultant who is involved personally or intimately with the client is not in a position to evaluate objectively between personal attractiveness and the consultant role.

The consultant is responsible for setting limits of personal involvement with the client. If the situation ever occurs that it is difficult to ignore sexual feelings to the point of making it impossible to interact at a professional level, the consultant should withdraw from the situation and arrange for a colleague to take over, if one is available.

Another point of sexual issue is that of sexism. Fenner (1980) defines sexism as "the label applied to the pervasive force of prejudice that assumes that certain characteristics or roles are appropriate to an individual or group of individuals solely on the basis of gender" (p. 171). Just as nursing has always been predominately a female field of practice, consultation has been a male one. Some clients will view the female consultant as weaker or more passive than her male counterpart. Some contracting and negotiating sessions early in the consulting relationship can be uncomfortable for the female consultant, especially on a one-to-one relationship with a male client or with an administrative group of male clients. It may be equally as uncomfortable for the male client or for the male consultant in the reversed situation. However, sexism in the selection of a consultant is a luxury that human survival can no longer afford or tolerate.

Consultation is concerned with esteem about one's abilities and achievements or with the self-confidence that characterizes the especially autonomous person. A consultant cannot function effectively without respect, and self-respect is the most important factor of all. It is not only respect for one's merits but respect for one's rights and one's own sexuality. Sexuality begins to make sense when it is viewed as part of the whole human experience. Knowledge about sexuality can give insight into one's inner and social self. The expression of sexuality is one of the ways in which one reaches out to others. For discussions of greater depth in the area of human sexuality, read Rosemary Hogans' *Human Sexuality: A Nursing Perspective* (1984) or the *Textbook of Human Sexuality for Nurses* by Robert Kolodny and associates (1979).

Truth-Telling and Promise-Keeping
The goal of consultation is to support and encourage client decision making. The consultant's image is frequently that of a trusted friend. Thus it is a serious issue when consultants misrepresent themselves and their qualifications and make unattainable or unrealistic promises about what they can do or cannot do for their clients. In the long run these violations of truth-telling and promise-keeping may do much harm. Certainly they disrupt the harmony of the consultant–client relationship and may be responsible for the complete failure of the consulting project.

Truth-telling and promise-keeping are seen as essential to the quality of human relationships. It is disturbing to see these fundamentals of human interaction compromised, minimized, and even eliminated supposedly in order to facilitate goal achievement. The consulting relationship should be one of trust and confidence. Any misrepresentation could result in a complete breakdown of trust in the consultant.

There are several areas that need to be considered under the category of truth-telling and promise-keeping. One area is that of deception. As a case in point, if someone introduces you as a consultant who knows a lot about graduate-level curriculum planning when in reality you do not, it would be deceiving the client to accept a contract under these circumstances. Conversely, there are some consulting experiences and other training techniques common to workshop and in-service education that involve deliberate deception—that is, withholding information for strategic teaching purposes. An example of this would be a planned session with a staff nursing group on communication techniques including abilities related to meaningful observation and listening. It might be part of the consultant's plan to use the first part of the session as an experiment in communication patterns. In this situation, deception—in the sense of the group not knowing what is happening—is part of the learning process. Even when the consultant does purposefully deceive workshop participants he or she must also be careful to undo the effects. Some structured experiences such as the example cited require that the consultant not discuss the goals before the activity. They must, however, be made explicit later.

Another area to consider is that of tangible reinforcers: payments in the form of kickbacks, bonuses, or bribes which raise ethical considerations that range from legal concerns about bribery to concerns about adverse behavioral effects. While the use of such reinforcers has been shown to change certain behaviors, their misuse is all too frequent. If, for example, the consultant has a personal interest in the selection of a particular nursing home by way of kickbacks or other financial interest, he or she may force the client or family selection by not giving due consideration to other sites. The consultant may even go so far as to promise follow-up supervision of the client in the nursing home knowing that any long-term contact will be improbable if not impossible. Such unethical activities hold out promises that the consultant has no intention or ability to fulfill.

Selling professional skills is another area that demands special consideration. The need for consultant accountability has already been emphasized in this chapter, and yet it needs reemphasis under truth-telling and promise-keeping. Regardless of the kind of consultation to be performed, consultants cannot ethically promise that they will be able to bring about certain types of outcomes. Nothing can be guaranteed when working with people. Consultants cannot promise what will happen as a result of their efforts, nor can consultants imply that people will be different when they leave or that the consultant will "set them free." In effect, the consultant cannot force unwilling clients to achieve any specific outcomes or learning.

SUMMARY

If there is a code of ethics for nurse consultants, it has much to do with self-awareness of one's own goals and values in relation to the client's goals and values. A conscious process of self-awareness by consultant and client makes them both more effective. By paying attention to patterns, values, strengths, and relationships, the consultant is able to appreciate the actions and feelings of the client. This awareness helps consultant and client work with each other instead of against each other, and contributes to the overall effectiveness of the consulting relationship.

Ill-considered value judgments cause as much trouble as any one other element in the consultant's dealings with clients. These value judgments include economic values (fee setting and padding expense accounts); moral values (autonomy, authority, coercion, manipulation, privacy, and sexuality); personal values (accountability, confidentiality, truth-telling, and promise-keeping); and many more.

The most difficult form of the ethical problem is the ethical dilemma—

the choice between two courses of action each of which would have unfortunate consequences. The consultant's notion of right and wrong and degrees of rightness and wrongness must come, in very large measure, from the moral values accepted by the group that compose the consultant's society—that is, from the ethical codes of professional nursing.

Thus the area of ethical responsibility for the consultant requires full consideration of ethical, moral, and value clarification processes, and a careful weighing of the probable consequences of intervention in the light of guiding values. It is not an easy matter to exercise such responsibility, partly because of ambiguity about which values should apply and partly because of difficulties of assessing the impact of intervention on the values chosen. Often moral ethical judgment rests heavily on a prediction about how a specific intervention will affect the client and other participants. It is important to remember that consultants are responsible for themselves and the effectiveness of their helping behavior; they are not directly responsible for the behavior or learning of others.

SELECTED REFERENCES

American Nurses' Association. *Code for nurses.* Kansas City, Mo.: ANA, 1976.

Curtis, L., & Flaherty, M. *Nursing ethics: Theories and pragmatics.* Bowie, Md.: Robert J. Brady, 1982.

Davis, A., & Aroskar, M. *Ethical dilemmas and nursing practice* (2nd ed.). New York: Appleton-Century-Crofts, 1983.

Donnelly, G., Mangal, A., & Sutterly, D. *The nursing system: Issues, ethics, and politics.* New York: Wiley, 1980.

Fenner, K. *Ethics and law in nursing: Professional perspectives.* New York: Wiley, 1980.

French, R. *The dynamics of health care.* New York: McGraw-Hill, 1974.

Hansen, J., Stevic, R., & Warner, R. *Counseling: Theory and process.* Boston: Allyn & Bacon, 1972.

Hogan, R. *Human sexuality: A nursing perspective* (2nd ed.). New York: Appleton-Century-Crofts, 1984.

Kolodny, R., Masters, W., Johnson, V., & Biggs, M. *Textbook of human sexuality for nurses.* Boston: Little, Brown, 1979.

Langford, T. *Managing and being managed.* Englewood Cliffs, N. J.: Prentice-Hall, 1981.

Lippitt, G. *Visualizing change.* La Jolla, Calif.: University Associates, 1973.

Mapes, T., & Zembaty, J. *Biomedical ethics.* New York: McGraw-Hill, 1980.

Patton, M. *Qualitative evaluation measures.* Beverly Hills, Calif.: Sage, 1980.

Pfeiffer, J., & Jones, J. Ethical considerations in consulting. In J. Jones & J. Pfeiffer (Eds.), *The 1977 annual handbook for group facilitators.* La Jolla, Calif.: University Associates, 1977, pp. 217–244.

Schulberg, H., Killilea, M. *The modern practice of community and mental health.* San Francisco: Jossey-Bass, 1982.

Simon, S. The search for values. *Edvance,* 1971, *1*(3).

Stein, J., & Su, P. *The Random House dictionary.* New York: Ballantine, 1980.

Sundeen, S., Stuart, G., Rankin, E., & Cohen, S. *Nurse–client interaction.* St. Louis: C.V. Mosby, 1981.

Taylor, P. *Principles of ethics.* Belmont, Calif.: Dickenson, 1975.

Warwick, D., & Kelman, H. Ethical issues in social interaction. In W. Bemis, K. Benne, R. Chin, & K. Cory (Eds.), *The planning of change.* New York: Holt, Rinehart & Winston, 1976, pp. 470–496.

Wolff, R. *In defense of anarchism.* New York: Harper & Row, 1976.

CHAPTER 12

Marketing, Negotiating, and Contracting

All consultants produce two basic operating functions—they produce a service and they market it.

B. Bradway and associates, 1982

This chapter is aimed primarily at the nurse who will go into consulting as a career function but is of equal value to those nurses who "use consultation" as a supplementary activity to their particular nursing role. The discussions in this chapter on marketing, negotiating, and contracting are designed to bridge the gap between having the desire and general skills needed to be a professional nurse consultant and having the knowledge of how to go about getting started. This is a "how-to" chapter that tells the nurse consultant how to market, negotiate, write contracts, and get on with the business of being a successful nurse consultant.

Not everyone doing consultation recognizes the need to be able to sell ideas and proposals to clients. This needs the creation of a market for one's services, promoting and selling one's expertise, preparing a written proposal for the client, negotiating that proposal, and signing a written contract. This type of marketing, negotiating, and contracting may not appeal to nurse consultants who somehow have fallen into a consulting role without ever planning for it and who depend on reputation alone to sell their consultant skills. These consultants wait, either patiently or impatiently, for clients to contact them. The notion that the consultant must develop a business orientation in order to continually and profitably grow as an individual entrepreneur did not pervade the consultant community until the 1970s (Bradway et al., 1982). Highly perceptive and astute consultants are realizing the need to approach the management and operation of consultation as a small business enterprise. Entire books, such as Ricardi and Dayani's *The Nurse Entrepreneur* (1982) and Mundinger's *Autonomy in Nursing* (1980) are now being published to assist nurses who wish to test new forms of autonomous nursing practice such as independent consultation. Hence a new philosophy and new thrust has evolved.

STRATEGIC PLANNING

Being an independent consultant calls for a certain amount of assertive activity on the part of the nurse consultant. With more and more nurses entering the consultant field, consulting will become more competitive and will depend on the sales ability of the consultant. The novice consultant must be highly visible and actively participate in national and regional nursing conferences, attend professional and related association meetings, and become an active member of professional consulting organizations such as the Nurse Consultants Association. Another source of exposure to consider is paying for listing (advertising) as a nurse consultant both in professional journals and with independent health consulting agencies. Whether or not a consultant has a chance to even be considered thus depends on effective marketing strategies, while obtaining and retaining positions depends on the ability to generate an attractive proposal and negotiate a contract acceptable to both consultant and client.

Strategic planning is an important process to implement prior to considering consultation as a major career endeavor. According to Bradway and associates (1982) there are four steps to strategic planning:

1. Developing an overall sense of direction—deciding where you want to go and when you want to get there.
2. Developing well-defined but realistic short- and long-term goals and objectives.
3. Developing a strategy for achieving goals and objectives. Answer the question: "How are you going to get there?"
4. Developing a method to anticipate changes that may alter or affect your decision to become a consultant. This approach requires developing a process to answer a "What if?" question. For example, what if you decide to do consultation on a full-time basis and cannot get enough consulting business to support yourself? Do you have alternatives available?

The whole process of planning for a career change or a reorientation in that career is characterized by risk and uncertainty, but effective planning allows for the flexibility and resilience that will be needed to minimize adverse events. There will always be risks, but for the creative consultant who has the initiative and personal characteristics needed to organize and be a successful consultant, the rewards are great.

THE CONSULTANT SPIRIT (KNOW YOURSELF)

Not all nurse experts will be, or can become, effective consultants. Insight into one's personality and potential is a fundamental requirement for success since the consultant role is a self-actuating and competitive one. The term "knowing yourself" is often used in the context of being able to recognize what characteristics one possesses that are associated with other successful consultants. For instance, not every nurse is the "type" to want to take the risk or to handle the hundreds of details necessary to start and firmly establish a consulting practice. A review of literature in this area, particularly that of Aiken (1982), Langford (1981), Kraus (1980), Ricardi and Dayani (1982), and Winston (1983), reveals a unique pattern of psychological and personality characteristics associated with successful entrepreneurs. These characteristics include:

1. Need for achievement, commitment to excellence, and desire to be a winner
2. Commitment to the task, energy, stick-to-itiveness, and willingness to assume responsibility
3. Aggressive ability to take on realistic tasks, but not gambling; preference for moderate risk
4. Alertness to opportunities and speed in seizing and converting them to advantage
5. Objective, realistic, unsentimental, business-like approach to solving problems
6. Stimulated by feedback on performance
7. Self-confident; optimistic in novel situations
8. Values money more as a measure of success than for wealth itself
9. Active managerial style, future-oriented, and a skillful organizer
10. Outstanding communication skills and social skills
11. Sensitive and receptive, able to analyze people quickly

These are important characteristics for any consultant. Consultation is not just a job but a continual challenge. The successful consultant thrives on pressure, loves adventure, likes helping people, and is outgoing and confident. It is possible to develop these characteristics, but remember that professional full-time or even part-time consultation is a demanding lifestyle.

MARKETING CONSULTANT SERVICES

The nurse who plans a career as a consultant needs to become thoroughly familiar with what is presently going on in the field of nursing consultation.

Guidelines on the role of the nurse consultant are published and updated periodically by the American Nurses' Association and the National League for Nursing. Nursing consultation involves practice, autonomy, authority (to determine the sole right of what the type of practice will be), and accountability. The responsibility that is inherent in this type of independent practice must be carefully weighed. In accepting the consultant role, the nurse also accepts the obligation to learn the craft of business management. No matter what form of consulting practice the nurse chooses, knowledge of marketing, negotiating, and contracting principles and procedures are a necessary part of the venture into consultation.

The search for ways to influence clients and sell ideas, proposals, budgets, and recommendations is clearly a new concern for most nurse consultants. Independent consultation is classified as a business enterprise—that is, it is an activity that satisfies human needs and wants by providing services for private profit. As such, the "selling" of consultant services requires the motivation for establishing, operating, and maintaining a business. And like any business, there are risks and rewards. The rewards of successful consulting are great; and the risks can be minimized through the planning of coherent business strategies, the first of which is marketing.

Developing a Marketing Strategy

Marketing is a plan of action. It involves all of the activities necessary to bring a "seller" (the consultant) and a "buyer" (the client) together. A marketing plan identifies the most promising business opportunities for the consultant. It outlines how to successfully penetrate, capture, and maintain desired consultant positions, and directs the performance of all activities that identify the flow of services from consultant to client (Chase & Barasch, 1977). In addition a marketing plan is also a communication tool that integrates all elements of the marketing mix (promotion, networking, advertising, financing, and public relations) into a single comprehensive program for coordinated action at all marketing levels. The plan specifies what services the consultant will offer, in what areas of the country the services will be offered, to what target population the services will be offered, and how the consultation process will be accomplished.

According to Chase and Barasch (1977) a good marketing plan:

1. Stimulates thinking to make better use of the consultant's resources.
2. Assigns responsibilities and schedules work.
3. Coordinates and unifies efforts.
4. Facilitates control and evaluation of results of all activities.
5. Creates awareness of obstacles to be overcome.
6. Identifies marketing opportunities.
7. Provides an authentic marketing information source for current and future reference.
8. Facilitates progressive advancement toward the consultant's goals.

Marketing does not have to be an elaborate procedure for the nurse consultant functioning in an independent or small team practice. It does, however, have to take into consideration the elements of strategy in planning specific consulting services to be offered, distribution areas of these services, promotional strategies to be used, and the setting of profitable and justified prices.

Planning Services

Consultants must have a clear concept of what they can do and specific guidelines for what they want to do. Many beginning consultants will hesitate to be so specific and will want to keep their service line broad for fear of turning away business or developing in a way that differs from their ultimate goals. There is a temptation for a beginning consultant to accept any project even if it is not in the consultant's line of work or specialty area. This type of approach can set a consultant up for disenchantment or even failure. In developing a service line, the consultant should not take assignments that may be questionable. For instance, the nurse consultant may be asked to consult with a group of cardiac intensive care nurses. If the client need involves the planning and giving of direct care and the consultant has only limited knowledge of this specialty function, it would risk the consultant's reputation to take the job, especially if there are better qualified consultants available.

Another example is a situation where a consultant is hired by hospital administration to act as a spy on staff members. Accepting an engagement out of fear that nothing better will be offered lowers self-esteem and diverts the consultant from becoming an acknowledged expert in a particular area. The consultant cannot be an expert at everything. It is better to become progressively more and more expert in a specific area. This will make both the job and marketing easier. According to Lant (1985), consultant specialization is both more marketable and more profitable.

Hence the key to increasing the chances of success is to keep focus on the area of expertise and to behave authentically and truthfully about one's abilities (both strengths and weaknesses) when defining and promoting service lines. Perhaps all failures cannot be avoided, but they can be minimized by a careful explanation of the scope of services offered.

Distribution and Promotional Strategies

Defining the distributional areas of a consulting service involves examination of the market for what you, as a consultant, have to offer. It requires a goodly amount of self-confidence and the ability to sell yourself and be able to strike out on your own in the business world. Most consultants will start consulting services in a fairly small geographical area, building a reputation locally before they branch out nationally or even internationally. A consultant in California, for example, may elect to restrict consultation to just the

Los Angeles or San Francisco area, since they are heavily populated areas with a reputation of extensive demand for nurse consultant services. On the other hand, a consultant based in Alabama or Mississippi might elect to extend the consultant distribution area to all of the southeastern states. It is important that such factors as travel, expense, time, and the facilitation of communications be carefully weighed before negotiating a contract.

Promotional strategies that involve personal selling, advertising, and networking must be blended together so as to communicate effectively with the potential market. Networking is an excellent way to begin. A consultant must develop a contact network. As Boone and Kurtz (1977), Downing (1971), Lant (1985), and Puetz and Gaithersburg (1983) point out, it is the most effective and least expensive marketing technique available and a consultant cannot operate successfully without it.

A contact network is a collection of acquaintances and other people who can facilitate the consultant's access to individuals, groups, and community organizations in need of consultant services. The greater the number of contacts in a consultant's network, the greater the chances of success.

The consulting agency is another type of agent go-between. The agency is a broker usually working on a commission and operating on a noncontinuous relationship of bringing individual consultant and client together to negotiate a contract. This arrangement is not the same as the independent consultant team in which the principal consultant may act primarily as the agent who organizes the team to fulfill certain contractual needs. In such an arrangement, the members of the consultant team are thoroughly familiar with one another and work together repeatedly. Joining consulting agencies or joint consulting practices is the new "supermarket of services" approach in which a consultant who specializes in a particular field becomes a member of a team of other specialists. Although these relationships can be complex, confusing, and competitive, they also have some advantages. For example, a multidisciplinary team can handle projects that an individual consultant cannot. It can also create unique combinations of skills. In addition, a team also has the advantage of being able to form and dissolve when needed.

Commercial advertising can be effective as a marketing tool if accomplished through professional channels. For a moderate fee (usually $30 to $100) a listing of consultant services can be placed in nursing education and nursing administration journals. The nurse consultant may even want to consider placing an ad in allied professional newspapers and journals. Another marketing possibility is the distribution of brochures by direct mail announcements. The brochures should include information about the consultant, areas of expertise, and examples of the type or types of consulting most frequently performed. Brochures are costly but can have a fairly high rate of response if directed to targeted persons of authority in specific organizational areas of interest to the consultant.

The beginning consultant in particular should take advantage of public exposure. Attend and present papers at nursing and interdisciplinary seminars and workshops and publish wherever possible. Recognition as an expert is the first step to marketing consulting services.

Fee Setting

As part of a market strategy, consultant fees should be set and standardized whenever possible. Consultant rates are usually competitive and depend heavily on reputation, years of experience, and specialization. Consultants should be familiar with the "going rate" for their professional field and specialty area. Consultant fees, usually in the range of $300 to $600 or more per day plus expenses, may appear to be very high, but remember that most consultants work only a few days at a time and must cover many of their own expenses such as secretarial help, telephone answering services, editing, printing, and copying. As a general rule, longer projects can be billed at a lower rate than short-term projects.

It is the responsibility of the consultant to state clearly, in the proposal to the prospective client, all expected expenses, and to set the daily consultant rate. The method of payment, whether it be hourly, daily, weekly, monthly, or only at the conclusion of the project, should also be stipulated in the proposed agreement.

In many of the longer and more involved consulting relationships, overall costs should not be finalized during the initial contact—for example, do not state specific terms such as five days a week at $500 per day when negotiating very vague, long-term projects. Rather, it is better to suggest subsequent stages that explain consultant involvement and tasks to be accomplished. Explain your tasks, stating for example that you will have a managerial role, gather information, write a report, or confer with involved personnel. If possible, be specific about the amount of time and cost for each step and arrange for interim payments at agreed-upon milestones. Do not underestimate your time, because you may find it difficult to change an estimate once the proposal has been made. Lant (1985) suggests that the consultant always allow a 20 percent time margin. On the other hand, do not inflate your time or cost requirement, as it may deter the client's acceptance of your proposal.

Another rule of thumb is to generally not charge for less than half a day. If you spend only two hours with a client, you charge for half a day. It is uncommon for consultants to charge hourly rates. Project fees are based on the number of days you expect to put into a project. If you expect a project will take five days, including your 20 percent leeway, charge five times your daily rate (Lant, 1985).

NEGOTIATING

Negotiating, the next phase of a business entrepreneurship, is defined by Cross (1969) as "the voluntary process of distributing the proceeds from cooperation" (p. 3)—that is, situations in which both consultant and client stand to benefit by reaching an agreement. Negotiation in this sense occurs in many nurse consultant–client contexts, from the one-to-one decisions on who performs what tasks to the complex negotiating that proceeds from marketing services through a multilevel consulting situation to the final goal outcome. For example, the negotiation of a fee is an important aspect of arriving at a clear treatment contract. Most clients have some knowledge of a consultant fee scale and more than likely are willing to pay the expected rate for the professional services they receive. If any disparity exists between the stated consultant fee and the client payment expectations, the client has the right to submit a request for a lower fee. The consultant can either reject this request or counter with an adjusted offer (for a discussion of unethical fee setting, see "Fee Setting" in Chapter 11).

In reality, consultants are concerned more with bargaining than with actual negotiating. Negotiating is viewed by many authors (Cross, 1967; Nierenberg, 1965; Pruitt, 1981; Rubin & Brown, 1975; Young, 1975) as being associated with the resolution of conflict, while bargaining is viewed more specifically as negotiation over the terms of a contract. It can be seen that the two terms are defined in nearly equivalent fashion. Whether the consultant is engaged in bargaining or in negotiating, at least one other party must be involved, the parties must be engaged in some form of transaction or interaction, and the purpose of this transaction must be to arrive at the settlement of some matter or issue. Given these defined similarities, the terms bargaining and negotiating are treated as synonymous throughout this chapter and book.

Functions of Negotiating

Negotiating is started on an equal basis—that is, the consultant has something "to sell" and the client is "buying." Much of the groundwork has already been covered by the time negotiations begin. By this time, the consultant has already been "marketed" to the client and the client situation has already been researched, to a degree, by the consultant.

It is not unusual for the client to enter the negotiating stage with a well-identified problem, since the problem has probably been a source of annoyance to the client for a period of time prior to seeking help. The client may even know what to do about the problem but often does not know how to implement the solution or needs an outside objective opinion.

Consequently, at this point successful negotiation depends on effective communication. By now both parties have their own identified needs and wants, and the satisfaction of those needs is the common denominator in negotiation. If consultant and client had no unsatisfied needs, negotiation would be an unnecessary task.

In general, for the consultant, the functions of negotiation are identifying client needs; developing specific agreements about roles, obligations, and privileges; and mediating change. These negotiation functions are discussed in the following sections.

Identifying Client Needs

The first interchange of communication between consultant and client is an exchange of information as well as ideas and concerns about the problem situation. The usual communication format used is that of interviewing, which will "seesaw" back and forth as the consultant tries to assess what the client is thinking and striving for while the client tries to determine how and whether or not the consultant can provide the help needed.

Effective interviewing by the consultant requires the ability to ask pertinent questions that will uncover the needs of the client. Nierenberg's *The Art of Negotiating* (1968) points out the importance of using only controllable questions—that is, those questions that will limit response. He compares the questioning ability of a good consultant to that of a lawyer in cross-examination who tries to stay away from types of questions where the answers are uncontrolled. In this context only questions that will uncover the needs of the client are used. As to the type of questions to employ, it may prove useful to recognize that most questions fall into five categories:

1. *General questions:* "What do you think?" "Why did you do it?" Such questions pose no limits, and therefore the answers are uncontrollable. These types of questions are useful tools in counseling but not consulting.
2. *Direct questions:* "Who can solve this problem?" "What have you done about it?" These questions contain limits, and therefore the answer is controllable within these limits.
3. *Leading questions:* "Isn't it a fact?" (answer controllable).
4. *Fact-finding questions:* Where?, Who?, When?, What? (answers controllable). How?, Why? (answers sometimes controllable).
5. *Opinion-seeking and validating questions:* Is it?, Do you think? (answers controllable) (Nierenberg, 1968).

The use of questions is a powerful negotiating tool and must be employed with discretion and judgment. The question determines the direction the conversation, argument, or bargaining will take. Effective questioning clearly determines client needs.

Development of Specific Agreements

Both consultant and client must concern themselves with multiple specific decisions that must take place during the negotiating stage. Examples are such things as negotiating for the environmental arrangements (office space, meeting rooms, and so on) needed for consulting activities, time commitments for both consultant and client, consultant fee arrangements, and the structuring (determination of limitations and authority) of the responsibilities of all parties involved in the consultation.

Mediation of Change

Change frequently emerges from negotiation. Personal needs of the consultant, the client, or both, may require modification before an effective collaborative relationship can be established, since it is not unusual for some conflict of interests to arise even in this early stage of a consulting relationship. Conflict can occur when the consultant comes on too strongly as an expert or too quickly presents ideas for change that the client isn't ready for. This type of consultant behavior may produce a backlash from the client, and an inconclusive struggle then develops until both parties, sensing the need for new structure and norms, agree to negotiate in an effort to develop a compromise or agreement acceptable to all involved.

Change, and adaptation to change, is constant in any consulting relationship. Change must be mediated by either consultant or client because until conflict differences are resolved, any discussions are likely to be fruitless. What is essential in such cases is a preliminary discussion and negotiation in which an agenda is developed that gives equal status to both the consultant's and client's main concerns. This can generally be accomplished by:

1. Maintaining a friendly, positive attitude
2. Listening attentively to the client
3. Being truthful on all points, and not exaggerating your experience or credentials
4. Not being critical
5. Being well-organized
6. Being flexible enough to meet the client halfway
7. Making sure both understand the terms of the contract
8. Knowing exactly what is expected of each other in the way of tasks to be accomplished

Negotiating Strategy

According to Pruitt (1981) the word "strategy" is considered in the negotiating context as comprising the techniques, tactics, and tools that the consultant uses to affect outcome during the process of negotiation. The particular strategies to be used depend on what the consultant seeks to gauge and measure and will differ greatly depending on the complexity and level of involvement in the consulting relationship. For example, negotiating strategies will not be the same for activities that originate with an individual client as they will be between groups and larger community organizations. Consider the following situations.

SITUATION A

A director of nursing, Ms. B., decides the time has come to standardize, and even possibly computerize, statements of nursing diagnoses in all nursing units of the hospital. After due consideration of the various courses of action open to her, Ms. B. decides to call in both a nursing consultant and a computer specialist.

SITUATION B

A group of staff nurses working in a cardiac intensive care unit propose a plan that could give even better nursing care to their patients. The plan involves an innovative approach to time scheduling for staffing. The solution of the problem would involve the input and coordination of not only the cardiac intensive care staff but of the supervisory and administrative staff as well. Subsequently, in order to get the input of all concerned and to coordinate activities, the hospital administrator agrees to hire a nurse consultant with administrative and managerial skills to study and implement this proposal.

SITUATION C

The nursing staff of a large city medical center complex has asked the hospital board for certain across-the-board increases in pay and fringe benefits. The board has refused to meet these demands, which it considers to be excessive. The staff then requests an American Nurses' Association consultant with expertise in labor negotiating to represent their groups in order to reach an agreement.

These three situations, diverse as they may appear, share a number of important features. Each illustrates a different level of negotiation or conflict, situation A being interpersonal, B intragroup, and C intergroup. Despite these differences, all three situations have the distinctive markings of a bargaining relationship, described by Rubin and Brown (1975) in terms of a number of prominent features:

1. At least two parties are involved. They may be individuals as in situation A, small groups as in B, or larger, more complex organizations or communities as in situation C.
2. The parties have a problem to solve with respect to one or more different issues. Where a single issue and a single client is at stake, negotiating strategies will on the whole be simpler and clearer to deal with. When addressing complex issues, the consultant should handle each separately in order of importance.
3. Regardless of the problem, negotiation must be approached as "true" collaboration or at least a temporary joining together in a special kind of voluntary relationship.
4. Activity in the relationship concerns the division or exchange of one or more specific resources and/or the resolution of one or more intangible issues among the parties or among those they represent.
5. The activity in complex consulting situations usually involves the presentation of proposals by one party, and evaluation of these by

the other, followed by concessions and counterproposals. The activity is thus sequential rather than simultaneous.

The ideal negotiating strategies for the consultant to use are those that will be most effective in the situation. The consultant must be the one to decide the approach strategies. These strategies depend on the desired outcome. Consultant and client must agree on whether (1) the concern of the consultation endeavor is to be put only upon the task of reaching the outcome itself (task-centered), (2) negotiation is needed to deal explicitly with the humanistic process of bringing about changes in client behavior that in turn bring about changes in an outcome (person-centered), or (3) focus should be upon attempts by either consultant or client to change some of the basic parameters of the situation (a combination of task-centered and person-centered approaches).

Negotiating in Conflict

Suppose that a nurse consultant is hired by a nursing school administrator to assist the faculty in developing a total revision of the school's nursing curriculum, and the faculty turned out to be in opposition to any proposed change. This type of conflict, one occasionally faced by nurse consultants, requires negotiations at two levels. Level one might be a relatively simple negotiation with school administration of mutually acceptable broad curriculum objectives and time and money considerations. Level two negotiations would come into play when the consultant begins to work directly with the faculty members involved. It is fairly obvious in this case that level two negotiations call for a much greater complexity of strategical techniques and tactics than level one.

Interests of various client levels should never be regarded as inherently opposed. Rather, Pruitt (1981) points out that the degree of divergence of interest at any time is a joint function of the parties' needs and the alternatives under consideration. It is quite possible for the parties to discover new alternatives that reduce or even eliminate a prior divergence of interest. For instance, in the example given the faculty and administration might find another curriculum (other than those under consideration) that combines the best points of the desired curriculum and provides benefit to both administration and faculty. Negotiations of this type call for complex integrative agreements—that is, ones in which "the participants all are satisfied with the outcomes and feel that they have gained as a result of the conflict" (Deutsch, 1973, p. 17). Negotiating strategies to effect a possible joint acceptance of a compromise curriculum would involve collaboration with the consultant in a problem-solving exercise weighing all possible alternatives as to their probability of success, value, and risk (as in Chapter 7, Fig. 17).

This is probably an oversimplification of the tactical approach that would be necessary to use in reducing resistance between administration and faculty, but the important point is the necessity for the consultant to create a truly collaborative relationship with all parties involved in the consulting endeavor. Agreement can only occur when all involved work together in search of a mutually acceptable answer.

In consulting situations where a great deal of conflict exists, there may appear to be periods of deadlock and renegotiation, with the bargainers exchanging concessions before they are able to engage in a problem-solving discussion that results in the emergence of a mutually prominent alternative. The consultant who knows and expects these stages of deadlock and coordination will not become easily discouraged or be over-anxious and force a progression that results in failure to achieve the goal. The theoretically prepared consultant will be a patient consultant and a successful one, since each negotiating stage will be expected and handled with competence.

CONTRACTING

If negotiation is a tool of human behavior, then contracting is a tool of decision making. During the contracting phase, decisions must be made about what the consultant "wants," what the consultant "needs," what the client "wants," and what the client "needs." It is essential for the establishment of a workable contract that both the consultant and the client have a clear idea of what the problem is, the purpose of the consultant's interventions, what the desired objectives are, and the means to be used to reach the identified goal. Furthermore, the consultant and the client must have the same goal—unless there is agreement, there is no point to a contract.

The consultant–client contract is an agreement to work toward stated objectives in a specified time. The use of a contractual agreement makes both the consultant and client accountable for the effort and time invested in their interaction. Responsibility for change is thus placed with both. If either party does not live up to the agreement, the other can request a reevaluation or termination of the contract.

Defining a Contract

A contract as defined in this book is a voluntary agreement between consultant and client that spells out the nature of their working relationships. A contract may be an oral agreement or a written document. To be legally enforceable, a contract must have the following characteristics:

1. The offer of the consultant and the acceptance of the offer by the client (or vice-versa) must be present.
2. Both parties must have the legal capacity to contract.
3. The contract must be for lawful purposes.
4. The expectations of both consultant and client must be specified in terms of tasks to be accomplished.
5. The value of services or monies involved must be stated.

6. The time limitations of the contract and renegotiation phases must be specified if needed (Bittle, 1980; Pruitt, 1981; Steckel, 1982; Ulschak, 1978).

A written contract lends an air of authenticity and importance to the relationship. "Contracts with external consultants are more often in writing because external consultants are trusted less than internal consultants, especially when it comes to money" (Block, 1981, p. 42). A written document signed by both parties will not only protect the consultant legally but will also help prevent misunderstandings. For example, a nurse consultant might have only a verbal agreement about work to be done in assisting a nursing staff to design a quality control system for the improvement of patient care on a particular hospital unit. Then suddenly, as the project nears fulfillment, the client (the director of nursing) states that the consultant promised to see to the implementation as well as the design of the system—a task to be accomplished within the same "set" fee structure. Without a valid written contract, it is the consultant's word against the client's word, and the consultant stands to lose the most—reputation, additional salary, and time. Even if the consultant finishes the job through the implementation stage, it is done under coercion, and neither consultant nor client is comfortable with the arrangement.

There may be occasions where a written contract is not feasible or warranted by the particular situation. In this case, an effective method to deal with a client in the absence of a formal contract would be for the consultant to write a letter of agreement summarizing the consultant's understanding of the verbal contract and including his or her expectations of the client as well as arrangements for fees and expenses. Giving this summary to the client in the presence of a witness or sending the letter to the client by registered mail provides acknowledgment of its receipt. Granted, this would be an unusual situation.

The Process of Contracting

The process of contracting cannot easily be differentiated from negotiation or other stages of the consulting process, since each is only a part of the whole. Contracting is the culmination or final agreement arrived at by both consultant and client. However, according to Ulschak (1978), there are two general approaches to contracting that can be useful as guidelines. One concentrates on establishing the relationship between the consultant and the client. The second approach attends to defining the relationship between the client and the problem.

In the first approach, the client's wants and needs for services are detailed along with the range of services the consultant is willing and able to provide. This period is a time of final decision about what the various parties involved want from each other and whether or not they are willing to enter into the relationship with all it entails. The client goal statement is included at this point.

In the second approach, contracting is a specific tool to specify, insofar as possible, the activities that will be needed to attain the goal. It details how the relationship will proceed and may involve not only the delineation of activities but such issues as time commitments, finances involved, or group maintenance issues as well.

In long-term contracting, the contract can be perceived as a dynamic process along a time line, as opposed to a single event. A long-term contract may be reopened for review and evaluation simply at the request of consultant or client for the purposes of redefining the relationship, to communicate desired changes, or to discuss possible termination of the relationship. The best approach to long-term contracting is the specification in the contract of review periods such as "In six weeks, twelve weeks, and six months, we will review the contract and update it."

Formulating the Contract

Every contract, written or verbal, is an extension of negotiation and should be clearly identified. Helvie (1981), Lant (1985), Merry and Allerhand (1977), and Stanhope and Lancaster (1984) all state that an operational definition of contracting should include the following components:

1. Joint exploration of the problem. There must be a clear statement of the problem which both parties agree upon
2. Establishment of objectives
3. Setting mutually agreed-upon goals
4. Joint exploration of resources to meet the goals
5. Development of a plan to meet the goals
6. Negotiation of a division of responsibility to meet the goals and agreed-upon action steps
7. Setting time limits to meet goals jointly
8. Determination of consultant fee payment schedule and client default clause
9. Establishment of procedures for evaluating progress toward goals Dates and times for such reviews should be specified
10. Setting procedures for modifying, negotiating, or terminating the contract

These components all involve joint collaborative planning at each step of the consulting process, negotiation at various stages, and division of responsibilities.

The contract format should be brief, direct, and almost conversational, while at the same time covering all necessary elements. Figure 28 shows an example of a short-form contract between a nurse consultant and a unit hospital staff. Figure 29 gives a long, more formal type of contract between a consultant and a school of nursing for the purpose of collaborating with faculty to implement a curriculum change.

I, *(consultant name)* will meet with the surgical nursing staff each Monday from 1 to 3 PM for the next four weeks *(January 3, 10, 17, 24)* for the designated purpose of educating staff to understand concepts and implementation of nursing process.

Hospital administration will provide a meeting place (physical and temporal arrangements) for the group. The fee agreed upon is *$300 per day.* No per-diem expenses are included but will be open to renegotiation if the client requires consultant time and services other than specified.

Date: _____

Consultant:	Client:
Signature: _____	Signature: _____
Name: _____	Name: _____
Address: _____	Address: _____
Phone: _____	Phone: _____

Figure 28. Short-form consulting contract.

Problem Areas in Contracting

The fundamental purpose of contracting is to organize cooperation for the purpose of accomplishing specific goals. If the atmosphere of cooperation is disrupted, or if either consultant or client becomes resentful or hostile toward the other, the consulting relationship may cease to be beneficial to either one of them.

One problem area that can lead to such a disruption can simply be the overstating by the consultant of the expectations of the results of the relationship. Cross (1969) found in his research that overstating one's payoff expectations will have the rather surprising result of operating to the consultant's own disadvantage. This usually results from inexperience, overconfidence, or simply an excessive desire on the part of the consultant to get the contract. This "oversell" is all too common in consulting practice. In the final analysis, when a consultant cannot deliver the services or results expected, the atmosphere of collaboration disappears and the consultant runs the risk of antagonizing and alienating the client completely. Both parties end up losing and the future reputation of the consultant is at stake.

A second problem area is concerned with the failure of the client to live up to contract promises. For example, a client may never have experienced a consultant relationship and may not understand, at the beginning, exactly what is involved in the total project. This is frequently the result of poor marketing and negotiating before contracting. It is important that the consultant be sensitive to the problems the client experiences with the contracting process. When the problems are identified correctly, contracting may be used to resolve or control them.

When contracting problems cannot be mutually solved through a prob-

This agreement entered into on (*date*) between (*consultant name*) and (*client name: School of Nursing*) for the purpose of providing consultant services to assist faculty in designing a graduate-level major in nursing consultation.

1. Client Goal. To implement a new graduate-level major in nursing consultation. This will include the following.
    1.1. Overall design of nursing consultation curriculum.
    1.2. Identification of specific courses.
    1.3. Details of course content.
    1.4. Clinical experience for students.
2. Services Provided by Consultant.
    2.1. Gather available data on programs already in existence in comparable schools of nursing.
    2.2. Initial meeting with administration and faculty to determine feasibility, fundability, marketing, and availability of faculty to teach, and exploration of clinical sites for student consulting experience.
    2.3. Meet with faculty to establish development priorities.
    2.4. Provide meeting and work schedules for general group meetings as well as individual meetings with faculty members.
    2.5. Collaborate with faculty to draft preliminary proposal for the new curriculum.
    2.6. Outline and distribute small group and individual work assignments on various aspects of the proposed curriculum.
    2.7. Maintain an "on-call" position with faculty for the duration of the contract.
    2.8. Encourage faculty to present their proposals and ideas. Summarize and draft their proposed curriculum concepts and content. Revise at general faculty meetings.
    2.9. Update drafts of curriculum content as revised. Distribute to faculty and administration.
    2.10. Repeat any or all aspects of the above until curriculum plan is accepted by faculty and administration.
    2.11. Weekly progress reports will be prepared for administration. Subsequent administrative contact as needed.
    2.12. Set dates and times for formative and summative evaluation reviews.
    2.13. Write a summary report of the project.
3. Responsibilities of Client to Consultant.
    3.1. Faculty and administration to attend all prearranged meetings.
    3.2. Faculty to carry out individual and small group assigned tasks.
    3.3. Faculty to keep consultant advised of progress and arrange for consultant collaboration where needed.
    3.4. Contract will be in force for a three-week period (15 working days). Renegotiable if further consultant time is needed.
4. Fees (including travel expenses).
    4.1. The consultant will be paid at the rate of $500 per day for a total of 15 working days (excluding Saturday and Sunday). Expenses to be paid additionally include:
        travel
        lodging
        long-distance phone calls when needed to fulfill contract
        food at $30 per diem
    4.2. Payment in full due upon completion of this contract including all per diem unless otherwise specified. Consultant will submit bills for all per-diem expenses.
    4.3. A service charge of 1.75 percent per month will be added in the event of any late payment or default.

Figure 29. Long-form consulting contract. (*cont.*)

4.4. In addition client agrees to pay all reasonable collection costs in the event of late payment or default.

5. General Conditions.

5.1. Consultant agrees to put forth maximum effort to achieve a comprehensive curriculum plan for a graduate-level nursing consultation major.

5.2. Client agrees to provide the consultant with office space, a meeting room, secretarial help, and duplicating services as well as access to school records pertinent to this contract.

5.3. Consultant agrees to seek client's approval on any major disbursement of more than $10 other than those designated in section 4.

Consultant: Client:

Signature: _____   Signature: _____

Name: _____   Name: _____

Address: _____   Address: _____

Phone: _____   Phone: _____

Figure 29. *(cont.)*

lem-solving and decision-making process, there are options available. For instance, a contract may simply be dissolved by mutual consent. Other cases may even proceed to the point of legal action, since the law does recognize it to be a duty to fulfill a written or verbal contract. When that duty is not performed by either the consultant or the client, the contract is breached, giving both parties certain legal resources.

SUMMARY

Planning and preparation are the keys to winning in the consulting business. The quality of the marketing, negotiating, and contracting done in a consulting endeavor is an accurate predictor of how the project will proceed. Consultants must be confident that their skills are congruent with what is needed by the clients and consonant with what they can deliver. To achieve congruence and consonance, clear goals must be set and a comprehensive assessment conducted to determine what is realistic and appropriate.

What does all this discussion of marketing, negotiating, and contracting mean to the nurse consultant? Cannot a nurse consultant function without being a "seller" of expert services? When we examine the answer to these questions closely, it becomes clear that any effective consulting requires considerable effort on the part of the consultant. The nurse consultant cannot help but "sell" services because, even if the client seeks out the consultant, negotiations will be needed to determine whether or not the particular consultant's skills are what the client needs.

Nurse consultants must alter their perceptions about the place of business management skills in their professional goals. Nursing consultation does not occur in isolation. From the discussions presented throughout this book, one can see how such diverse factors as communication, human relationships, problem solving, decision making, change, ethics, marketing, negotiating, and contracting all have an impact on consultant and client behavior.

The tendency is for nurse consultants to find themselves isolated from other types of consultants because of working specifically in the nurse-related field. Indeed, it is not unusual for nurse consultants to view themselves as isolated from even other nurses when it comes to areas of function. Much of this isolation behavior results from the lack of viewing consultation itself as a combined professional and business skill. If consultants seek profit, growth, and survival, they must do so by entering the business world and creating and offering services in the open market where the client either buys or does not buy.

This is what professional nursing consultation is really all about: not merely to develop a "sell" of expertise, but to develop a process of integrated strategies and market behaviors—via promotion, pricing, and logistical decisions—that will result in satisfying, productive consulting experiences.

SELECTED REFERENCES

Aiken, L. *Nursing opportunities in the 1980s: Crises, opportunities, challenge.* Philadelphia: Lippincott, 1982.

Bell, C., & Nadler, L. *Clients and consultants.* Houston: Gulf Publishing Company, 1985.

Bittle, L. *Business in action.* New York: McGraw-Hill, 1980.

Block, P. *Flawless consulting: A guide to getting your expertise used.* San Diego: Distributed by University Associates, 1981.

Boone, L., & Kurtz, D. *Contemporary marketing.* Hinsdale, Ill.: Dryden Press, 1977.

Bradway, B., Frenzel, M., & Pritchard, R. *Strategic marketing: A handbook for entrepreneurs and managers.* Reading, Mass.: Addison-Wesley, 1982.

Chase, C., & Barasch, K. *Marketing problem-solver.* Radnor, Pa.: Chilton, 1977.

Cross, J. *The economics of bargaining.* New York: Basic Books, 1969.

Deutsch, M. *The resolution of conflict: Constructive and destructive processes.* New Haven: Yale University Press, 1973.

Downing, G. *Basic marketing: A strategic systems approach.* Columbus: Chas. E. Merrill, 1971.

Helvie, C. *Community health nursing: Theory and practice.* Philadelphia: Harper & Row, 1981.

Kraus, R. *Information counseling and consulting for the organization.* Washington, D.C.: U.S. Dept. Health and Human Services, National Institute of Education, 1980.

Langford, T. *Managing and being managed.* Englewood Cliffs, N.J.: Prentice-Hall, 1981.

Lant, J. *The consultant's kit: Establishing and operating your successful consulting business* (2nd ed.). Cambridge, Mass.: JLA Publications, 1985.

Merry, U., & Allerhand, M. *Developing teams and organizations.* Reading, Mass.: Addison-Wesley, 1977.

Mundinger, M. *Autonomy in nursing.* Germantown, Md.: Aspen Systems Corporation, 1980.

Nierenberg, G. *The art of negotiating.* New York: Hawthorne Books, 1968.

Pruitt, D. *Negotiation behavior.* New York: Academic Press, 1981.

Puetz, B., & Gaithersburg, M. *Strategies for success: Networking for nurses.* Rockville, Md.: Aspen Systems Corporation, 1983.

Ricardi, B., & Dayani, E. *The nurse entrepreneur.* Reston, Va.: Reston Publishing Company, 1982.

Rubin, J., & Brown, B. *The social psychology of bargaining and negotiation.* New York: Academic Press, 1975.

Stanhope, M., & Lancaster, J. *Community health nursing.* St. Louis: C.V. Mosby, 1984.

Steckel, S. *Patient contracting.* Norwalk, Conn.: Appleton-Century-Crofts, 1982.

Ulschak, F. Contracting: A process and a tool. In J. Pfeiffer & J. Jones (Eds.), *The 1978 annual handbook for group facilitators.* La Jolla, Calif.: University Associates, 1978.

Winston, S. *The organized executive: New ways to manage time, paper and people.* New York: W. W. Norton & Co., 1983.

Young, O. *Bargaining.* Chicago: University of Illinois Press, 1975.

CHAPTER 13

The Final Note: A Blueprint for the Nurse Consultant

As a rule . . . he (or she) who has the most information will have the greatest success in life.

Benjamin Disraeli

As a final summary on how to use and adopt the ideas in this book, this chapter offers a set of numerically ordered guidelines. These guidelines provide the nurse consultant with a handy reference, in the format of a checklist, of the essential steps and consultant tasks that comprise the total consulting process.

1. Remember that there are as many individualistic approaches to consulting as there are consultants. It is a field that many nurse experts find themselves a part of because of job expectations, the need for supplementary money, or simply the demand of client cries for help.
2. Prepare yourself educationally, being especially cognizant of the need for strength in the areas of psychology, behavioral psychology, interpersonal and intragroup dynamics, role theory, change theory, social change, decision making, organizational development methods, scientific methodology, research, and especially business management skills.
3. Define a specialty area. You must start with a clear concept of the services you intend to offer. Specialization in a particular area makes you more marketable.

4. Plan ahead. Planning and preparation are the keys to winning in the consultant business. Continually examine your role and values as a consultant—this is critical both in terms of your personal growth and your professional development.
5. Focus on developing the knowledge, skills, and judgment needed to be a successful consultant. Use the consulting process as presented in Part II, Chapters 4 through 7. In this way you will develop a conceptual framework that provides you with a valid model of consultant functioning.
6. Recognize that there may be a need to deviate from a "set" consulting process and change your consulting style as demanded by the situation. Flexibility is the mark of a well-prepared and experienced consultant.
7. Gain experience first as a part-time consultant, working wherever possible as a member of a consulting team. Don't hesitate to let it be known that you are available for work as a consultant.
8. When you are ready to consider consultation as a major activity, do so effectively by using the principles and concepts of marketing and business management, paying attention to identifying and researching your market environment.
9. Identify your specialty field and preferred practice areas. Internalize the process of problem identification, especially concerning those problems for which you may have a solution. Develop your specialty field to the maximum.
10. Join the Nurse Consultants Association and other professional and nonprofessional organizations that you feel may give you some exposure to potential clients. Subscribe to journals related to your specialty area and watch them carefully for potential consultant activities in your field. *Nursing Success Today* (a journal) and *The Nurse Entrepreneur's Exchange* (a newsletter) are two periodicals that focus on the advancement of nurses in extended career endeavors.
11. Write and publish as many articles and offer as many workshop presentations as you can work into your schedule. Talk or write to the leaders in nursing consultation and learn from them.
12. You cannot succeed without a contact network of acquaintances and people who can facilitate your access to clients that need your help. Don't forget to include family, current colleagues, professional groups, civic groups, and religious groups. Tell everyone what you are doing, giving them your business card. Networking is a major marketing technique.
13. Sell your expertise. Advertise in professional newsletters and journals. Have a brochure professionally designed and printed describing your service line and qualifications. The brochure should not quote prices—leave this area open for negotiation. Make sure that

your name, address, and telephone number are on the outer panel or cover of the brochure. Mail brochures to potential clients.

14. If you cannot afford expensive advertising, volunteer your consulting services to some organization on a specific task in exchange for a reference. If possible, make sure that it is a prestigious organization such as the federal government (a grant project, for example), the American Red Cross, your state nurses' association, or a large medical center.

15. When you are approached with a consulting proposal, respond with interest and ask for specific details of the purpose and project. Respond politely even to those you reject. Elicit the client's expectations of you. Do not take assignments immediately if you have any reservations about the circumstances involved. Rather, respond with a promise to send a proposal to make sure that your experience will fit their needs and set up a future contact date with them. Postpone questions regarding time involvement, fees, and specific functions until the next meeting. Then check with others who might know the problem situation before final contracting. Say no to any project that in your judgment has less than a fifty-fifty chance of success.

16. Send a proposal to the client following the initial interview. (Some consulting inquiries are made by mail and proposals are sent before the interview takes place.) A proposal is a preliminary plan of action that identifies your expertise in the specified area of need. Include what you propose to do for the client, what you want from the client, and how much time, energy, and commitment you are prepared to put into a helping relationship. The proposal in the form of a letter or memorandum should be typed neatly and professionally. It should be clear and concise.

17. Generally, negotiations for a contract follow the submission of a proposal. A contract, if at all possible, should be a written document. Oral agreements are legally valid but it will help prevent misunderstandings to have details in writing. Chapter 12 includes samples of both short- and long-form contracts with detailed explanations.

    Most of your contracts should contain these elements:
    • Objectives of the project
    • Your role in the project
    • The client's role in the project
    • The product you will deliver
    • Time schedule
    • Fee schedule
    • Confidentiality acknowledgement

18. Once the contract has been signed, arrange a meeting with the client to clarify any unanswered issues and to make sure that both

you and the client have identified the problem correctly and have the same desired outcomes. Settle all the details involved in the project.

19. One of the most important criteria for predicting the likelihood that a useful and successful association will result is the initial relationship between you and the client. Take the time to build an appreciation, acceptance, and understanding of one another. Take no steps without the client's informed consent.

20. Keep in mind that the optimal consulting relationship is based on trust and respect. From the standpoint of effective consultation your relationship with the client should meet two criteria: the job or project must be accomplished effectively, and both you and the client should grow and develop.

21. Once the consulting relationship is established, assist the client to move toward exploration of the specific problem. It may be necessary for you to obtain additional information to help the client isolate and identify the problem.

22. The consulting process is a set of activities on your part that help the client to perceive, understand, and act upon events which occur in his or her environment. Remember that consulting is collaborating.

23. The consulting process moves in sequential stages from entry, goal setting, problem solving and decision making to termination of the consulting relationship. Do not proceed to the next step without completing the one you are presently in.

24. During the goal-getting stage three major tasks are paramount: a tentative goal must be specified, the consulting mission must be clarified, and there must be a determination of the final goal.

25. Keep basic concern focused on the task or goal to be accomplished rather than on specific individuals or groups. Consultation is a task-oriented process.

26. Continue to nurture a positive relationship with the client. Include the client as a partner wherever possible (if so desired by the client). Deal with resistance as it arises, even if it does not affect results.

27. Use everyday language. Avoid nursing jargon unless working with a nurse or nursing-group client. Words used by the consultant should facilitate the transfer of knowledge, not hinder it.

28. Treat the client's ideas on setting and meeting goals as valid and relevant information. Remember you are a facilitator, not the producer or decision-maker.

29. Operate always to expand and maximize the range of available information and possible alternatives so that the client can make the final decisions with as much data as possible.

30. Identify resources of potential people, materials, or systems available that may need to be deployed for problem solving.

31. Support and encourage the client toward realistic development of how things should be done. It is often helpful to show the client how others have resolved similar problems and to demonstrate the results they achieved.

32. When client problems are of a multiple and involved nature, keep simplifying, narrowing, and reducing the list of subgoals and alternative choices so that they focus more and more on the steps the client can take. Eliminate unnecessary and unwieldy subgoals.

33. Work toward value clarification and explain systematic and preventive intervention.

34. Provide the client with techniques that will focus his or her activities on the desired goal. Use of the models shown in Figures 14 and 16 (Chapter 7) provides a very sophisticated and workable methodology to assist effective client problem solving, decision making, and development of a plan of action.

35. A plan of action tells all parties involved what to do, when, how, who is responsible, and the outcomes expected. The decision for intervention now belongs to the client, the best decision being the alternative foremost on the problem-solving ranking.

36. Assist the client to develop the necessary skills to increase the probability of success. Another element of this focus is the continued importance of your support. Praise the client for small successes and the attainment of subgoals. The major client motivation for continuing effort comes from frequent expressions of successful movement toward the final goal.

37. Initiate "stop sessions" in which you both take a look at the progress and review process issues. This helps to ensure optimal focus of energy on the tasks yet to be accomplished. Periodic formative evaluation is vital to process success.

38. The continuing assessment of consequences of action is a crucial element of your role during the action-taking stage.

39. At all times your focus should be on the identification of things that tend to impede movement toward the desired outcome and those things that facilitate such movement. All client discussions must be analyzed as to their power to inhibit or facilitate goal achievement.

40. It may at times become necessary to revise action and mobilize additional resources whenever blockages and resistance to planned change occur. The model for viewing and analyzing the driving and restraining forces provided in Chapter 7 (see Fig. 14) enables you and the client to analyze the positive and negative forces inhibiting constructive client action.

41. An effective way to deal with a restraining or resistive force is to convert it to a driving or helping force.

42. Throughout the various stages of the consulting process, intervene by initiating intervention strategies as needed.

43. Intervention strategies are special consultant skills that support the client's change efforts. The intervention strategies of receiving, informing, energizing, and reflecting can and do occur at any time in the consulting process.

44. The ending of a consulting project (termination) should be viewed as a legitimate stage of the consulting relationship and another opportunity for consultant and client learning. The goal for the termination stage is to make sure that the client leaves the transaction with an appropriate sense of optimism and direction.

45. Like all other consulting activities, evaluation is not confined to the termination stage. Rather, it is a constant process of feedback sessions that monitor ongoing activities (process or formative evaluation), culminating with the measuring of final outcomes (outcome or summative evaluation).

46. Separation should be a mutually satisfying termination of the relationship. It helps to remember that your objective is for the client to be able to do independently that which he or she was initially dependent on you to accomplish.

The Nurse Consultant's Library: General Books on How to Establish Your Consulting Business

The following books are excellent references for the practicing nurse consultant.

1. Bell, C., & Nadler, L. *Clients and consultants*. Houston: Gulf Publishing Company, 1985.
2. Bermont, H. *How to become a successful consultant in your own field*. Available from The Consultant's Library, 815 15th Street N.W., Washington, D.C. 20005.
3. ———. *The successful consultant's guide to fee setting*. Available from The Consultant's Library, 815 15th Street N.W., Washington, D.C. 20005.
4. ———. *The successful consultant's guide to writing proposals and reports*. Available from The Consultant's Library, 815 15th Street N.W., Washington, D.C. 20005.
5. ———. *The successful consultant's guide to winning government contracts*. Available from The Consultant's Library, 815 15th Street N.W., Washington, D.C. 20005.
6. ———. *The successful consultant's guide to authoring, publishing, and lecturing*. Available from The Consultant's Library, 815 15th Street N.W., Washington, D.C. 20005.
7. Block, P. *Flawless consulting: A guide to getting your expertise used*. Available from University Associates, 8517 Production Avenue, San Diego, Calif. 92126.
8. Coffin, R. *The negotiator*. Available from the American Management Association, New York.
9. Goldstein, L. *Consulting with human service systems*. Available from Addison-Wesley, Reading, Mass.
10. Kinlaw, D. *Helping skills*. A facilitator's package, which consists of a guide and

a cassette tape that provide assistance for developing helping skills. Available from University Associates, 8517 Production Avenue, P.O. Box 26240, San Diego, Calif. 92126.

11. Lant, J. *Money talks: The complete guide to creating profitable workshops and seminars in any field.* Available from JLA Publishing Company, 50 Follen Street, Suite 507, Cambridge, Mass. 02138.

12. ———. *The consultant's kit: Establishing and operating your successful consulting business.* Available from JLA Publishing Company, 50 Follen Street, Suite 507, Cambridge, Mass. 02138.

13. ———. *The unabashed self-promoter's guide: What every man, woman, child and organization needs to know about exploiting the media.* Available from JLA Publishing Company, 50 Follen Street, Suite 507, Cambridge, Mass. 02138.

14. Ricardi, B., & Dayani, E. *The nurse entrepreneur.* Reston Publishing Company, Reston, Va. 22090.

15. Wasserman, P., & McClear, J. *Consultants and consulting organizations directory.* Available from Gale Research Company, Book Tower, Detroit, Mich. 48226.

16. Winston, S. *The organized executive: New ways to manage time, paper and people.* W. W. Norton & Co., 500 Fifth Avenue, New York, N.Y. 10110.

Index

Italicized page numbers refer to figures and tables